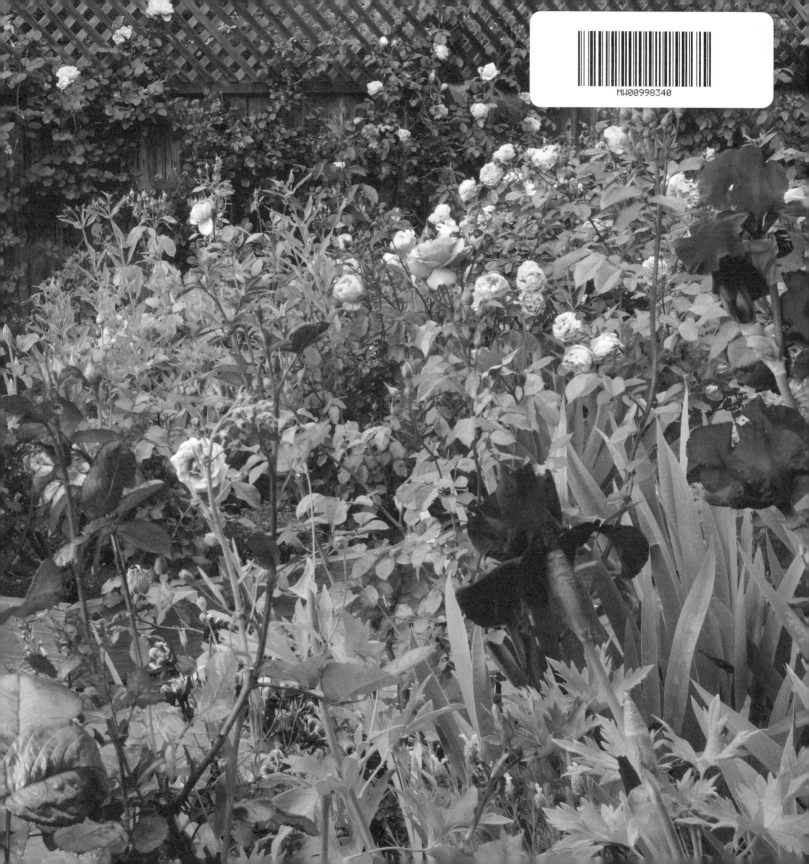

The Museum
of Scent

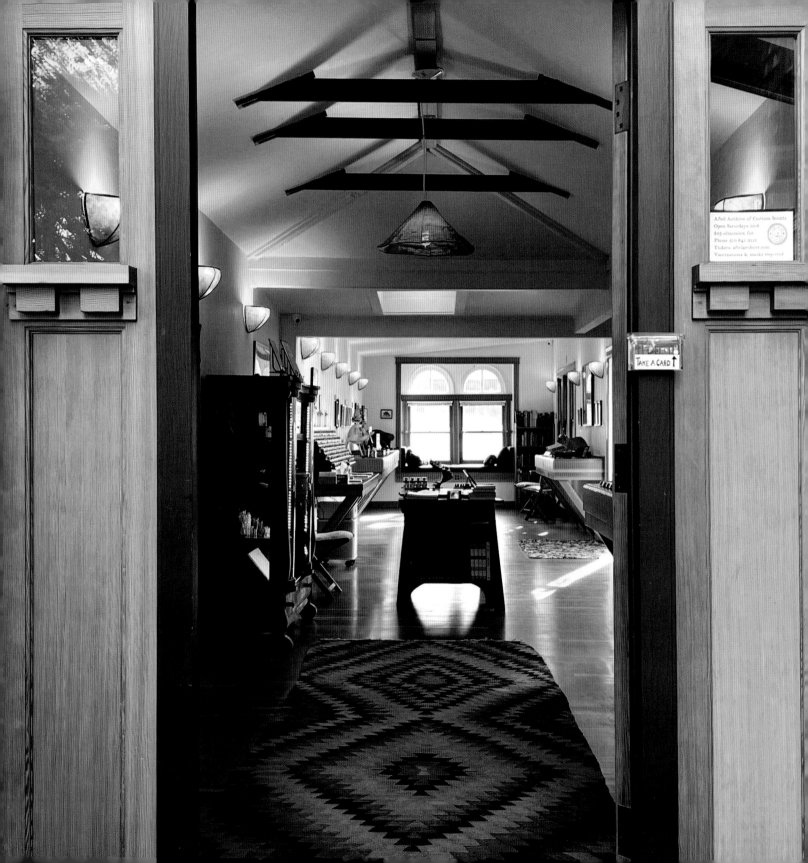

The Museum of Scent

Exploring the Curious & Wondrous World of Fragrance

Written & illustrated by
Mandy Aftel

Photography by Foster Curry

Foreword by
Dr. Clarissa Pinkola Estés Reyés

Abbeville Press
New York   London

For Foster and Devon

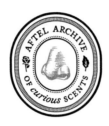

Contents

Foreword

Mandy Aftel: Mistress of Fragrances

I'd begin by gently offering that, over the decades, being in my seventy-eighth year on Earth, rarely do I see truly original manuscripts. Many works, published or not, are derivative: like a moderate to weak broth that is like "the water of the water" that the duck ran through.

However, this work by Mandy Aftel, internationally recognized parfumier, is a true original—a rarest of rare legacy volume. This book was created by a beautiful elder who is a polymath: meaning, a highly unique person of multiple modern and old ways of knowing.

Let us count those ways: Mandy Aftel is a sensitive observer, thus a clear and poetic writer. Inside this work, too, are her tender colorings of old botanical prints. These now carry her graceful and lyric choices of chromas.

This work is not written in the usual manner of some, that is, to "sit down and write something," but rather, knowing Mandycita, it was conceived, incubated, and born from the godly DNA of a woman scientist—who knows as much about fragrance molecules as she knows about the base notes of musks.

Many years ago, my grandson and I were honored to be her students in perfumerie first and second levels, working toward mastery. As a poet, my heart spun gold and nearly fainted, as I heard her speak so softly of "angel water"—a combination of scents—of attar, of civet, of cassolettes, tiny boxes with perforations to subtly scent the air—

and so many more striking phrasings that carried ancient history, the mind-bending sensual, the mysteries of the sexual, the mystical hauntings of fragrances remembered—not one-inch-deep trivia, but ever-expanding full body, mind, heart, spirit, and soul immersion in and through scent.

If one were to have a guide/teacher of wisdom in the *Paradiso*, there is none more finely tuned than the author of *The Museum of Scent*. . . . Her ways with conjuring and combining scents can lift, show, heal, help, delight truly . . . as plant medicine is wont to do—humanity being ensorceled by striking and subtle natural scents alone, since time out of mind.

I can aver unequivocally that she is a fierce engineer of tastes, scents, and fragrances—like new-mown hay, and newborn baby, and ceremonial cacao. La Señora Aftel is also a mathematician in her own right, creating her vast libraries of formulae with a fine-tuned sense of the music inside each taste, fragrance.

She is a lifelong learner with a library that stretches back, near it seems, to the beginning of Chinese printing plates: regarding also the heavens to be found, in how Creator laid down scent in layer upon layer, into everything. Everything, truly. Red sand, fog, natural skin scent, many different kinds of rain.

She is an inventor and also above all, for we know her in depth, she is that rare being: A holy person who does not crow "Me me me, I am great!" but shelters and encourages her students to *make her students* great.

La Diosa y El Dio te bendigan! May all of Greater and Creator bless and guide all seekers into fullest True Self, fullest health, and meaningful callings, via the many often astonishing sensory "ways of knowledge" we were all born with—

related to ingestion and immersion in the natural gifts given to us since the beginning of time—from the earth, the weather, the plants, the creatures, and more.

And to that progress: The Mistress of Fragrances, Mandy Aftel's *dons* and talents are now resting in your hands in this magical tome—that, I deeply sense and hope, will bless you time and again. . . .

—Dr. Clarissa Pinkola Estés Reyés

Dr. Clarissa Pinkola Estés Reyés, author: Women Who Run with the Wolves: Myths and Stories of the Wild Woman Archetype, *published in forty-two languages. Forthcoming work:* La Curandera, Walking in Two Worlds, *from Texas A&M University Press.*

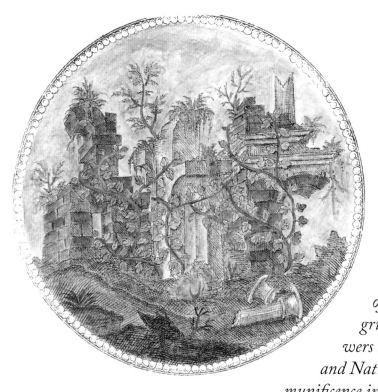

I
Aromatic Atlantis

In all countries, . . . in the religious festivals of all creeds, and on all occasions whether of grief or rejoicing, the scented attractions of flowers and plants possess an important significance, and Nature seems to have been most bountiful in her munificence in scattering these odiferous treasures throughout our world, to give cheerfulness to the earth and happiness to its inhabitants.

—Donald MacDonald, *Sweet Scented Flowers and Fragrant Leaves*, 1895

I've spent a lot of my adult life working in a world that you can't see—a world full of smells. These invisible aromas are all part of the extraordinary lineage of scent that reaches back to the beginnings of human culture and is entwined with the earliest history of medicine, cuisine, sexuality, adornment, and worship. As an artisanal perfumer who works with extraordinary aromatic ingredients from all over, I venture deep into this fragrant world every day. I fell in love with botanical essences thirty years ago and discovered that I had a knack for blending them to make perfume. I set up my own perfume business and gradually developed a following for my artisanal fragrances. It was almost enough for me just to enjoy searching for and using the best essences

I could find in the world. But I was also driven to know their origins: where these amazing materials came from, who used them, how, and what for. I wanted to learn the stories of how they fit into our lives. In this book, you can see each essence's particular color, see a hand-colored antique woodcut of the magnificent plant from which it was extracted, and learn about its lore and aromatic properties and uses.

The centerpiece of my life is the plant extracts, the essential oils— they are the thread that runs through my work. From medicine to spirituality, perfume, and aromatherapy, these essences not only represent the beauty of the natural world, but offer a window into our history. These amazing natural essences have always been a gateway into the beauty of nature—beauty that has inspired so many artists and creators. People fell in love with these essences and studied, revered, examined, and caressed them; they also wrote about them and drew, painted, and photographed them. You can see their passion for aromatic essences in the paper trail they left behind!

When I first became interested in this world, I had no idea how infinite the learning and pleasure could be. Each door opened out into another beautiful room. I began this journey into scent by collecting antique books about perfumery. My intention was simply to educate myself, but before long I was enchanted by their luscious interweaving of botany, history, religious customs, beauty, and herbal medicine. As I got to know the rare book dealers, I discovered which of them sometimes also had astonishingly beautiful postcards depicting the harvesting of

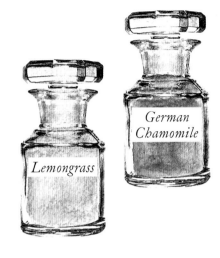

Lemongrass

German Chamomile

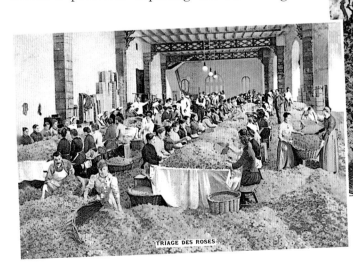

TRIAGE DES ROSES

Cueillette des Violettes

9   AROMATIC ATLANTIS

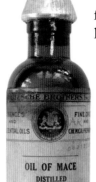

OIL OF MACE
DISTILLED

NEW YORK

flowers and other aspects of old perfume traditions, hand-tinted like paintings. Over time I began to collect them as well.

Then one day in a local antique store, I spotted a mysterious bottle of antique essential oil with a faded yellowed label, and bought it. I consulted with a friend who was a professional perfumer at a big fragrance house, and he told me my find was so old as to be useless, and I should dump the contents right down the drain. But when I lifted its battered metal neck cover, loosened the cork, and smelled, I was enveloped by the most exquisite, rich, multilayered aroma I had ever encountered. I was hooked! I continued to collect more and more antique oils.

I found that same sense of discovery and newness in the magnificent old books about herbs—"herbals," with their detailed renderings of the beauteous world of plants in woodcuts and copper engravings. These images identified each plant individually, leaf by leaf. One of the most famous herbals ever was *Theatrum Botanicum*—truly a Theater of Plants with over 4,000 mostly medicinal varieties, divided into seventeen "tribes" like "cooling herbs" and "venomous plants and their counter poisons." This massive volume includes some 2,700 woodcuts of plants, executed by several different artists. I painted the black-and-white woodcuts from the *Theatrum* to illustrate the plants whose essences are featured in *The Museum of Scent*. Here you can see the original woodcut of oakmoss and the watercolor I painted of it.

Because the plants permeated everything from medicine to sexuality, food to bathing, there was a sense of their pervasiveness in one's life. One thing leads to another: recipes for perfumes lead to recipes for essential oil–laden drinks; paintings of plant-gathering lead

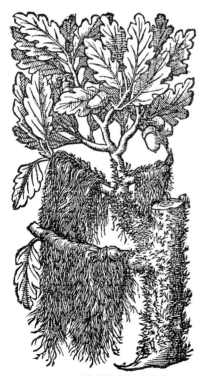

813.—OAK WITH MOSS.

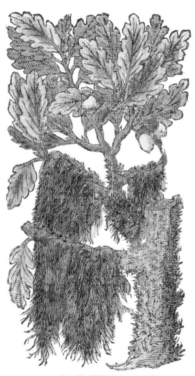

813.—OAK WITH MOSS.

to moody photographs of the various processes of extracting essences from plants. I fell into a whole and complete aromatic world that most people know nothing about. I was astonished at the workmanship and the beauty inherent in the old engraved emblems, the pomanders, the patch boxes. All of it reflected how precious beauty was in people's lives and how these essences inspired them—*inspire* literally means "to breathe in." Using them drop by drop to make my perfumes, I too revered the essences for the beauty they brought to everything I made.

It was like uncovering the lost continent of Atlantis, discovered bit by bit with my imagination helping put the pieces together. I felt like I had embarked on a lifelong treasure hunt, where every single thing I found was incredibly beautiful and special, with a pulsating newness. Fragments of this lost world—based on the importance *and* the beauty of natural aromatics—are still around now. I found so many things I had never known before, nor seen documented anywhere. Each aromatic treasure felt personal to me, but at the same time archetypal, even sacred, and rarely easy to get.

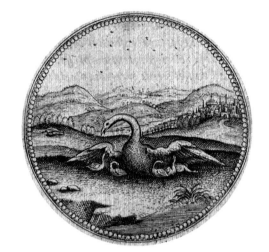

One of my rarest finds was the original book of emblems, *Symbolorum et Emblematum* (published in four parts between 1590 and 1604, and later issued as a single volume). This was the very first botanical emblem book, and one of the earliest uses of engraved intaglio plates for plant and animal illustrations—an ideal marriage of an herbal and a bestiary. Each picture, illustrating the world of plants, animals, and symbols, is a small narrative about life. Here you can see an original black-and-white emblem from the *Symbolorum* and my watercolor painting of it. Each chapter of *The Museum of Scent* starts with one of these hand-colored emblems, chosen to convey the chapter's meaning in a *sui generis* image.

I like to visit the tiny museums of the Gold Rush in the tiny towns of the Gold Country of California, a few hours north of me. In one of them, the idea came to me that I, too, could make my own little museum of the things that I had collected. After many years of being immersed in this aromatic world, it was time to share it as a museum—and, of course, as a book! Every item in this book lives in the Aftel Archive of Curious Scents.

This book is about a world apart from reality, where the reader can experience the truth I have learned: It's not that the world of scent contains these objects so much as they contain the world. This world kindles a sense of shared humanity that transcends the boundaries of culture and travels down through the eras. It shakes us out of our usual way of responding to the modern world, as a lifeless place; the universe of aromatics has the power to vivify our very being, to remind us of the difference between what is alive and what merely exists. It opens up an imaginative and creative place where people discover not only more about the world but more about themselves. It propagates an experience that's transporting, imaginative, and personal, where the reader's own imagination can be sparked by the beauty, weirdness, and universal pull of aromatic materials and artifacts, and by the charged and often elusive and indefinable memories and emotions they bring forth. The world of curious scents leaves you transformed. You start in one place and come out enriched, stimulated, with a greater sense of possibility, like when you've taken a walk in the forest or meditated—you come back more whole.

How does one convey the world of fragrance in a book, without anything to smell (except the bookmark inside the back cover)? *The Museum of Scent* is full of reveries designed to stir the imagination, to spark personal connections between the reader and the words and images on the page. The images themselves occupy this demiworld.

My hope for this book is not so much that it be understood, but that it reverberate. It is an invitation to an awareness of ways of being that we have forgotten. The richness and depth of experience that are contained within aromatic materials—how they were discovered, unlocked, refined, handed down from generation to generation, and transported from place to place—can be an endless source of inspiration. While modern society tries to transform us into ghosts or robots, we can instead feel alive and engaged with nature. Come enter this world!

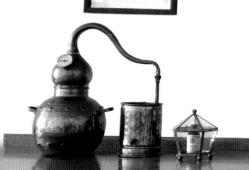

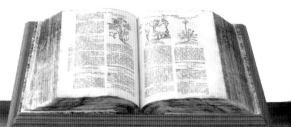

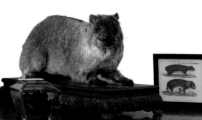

2 Getting to the Essence

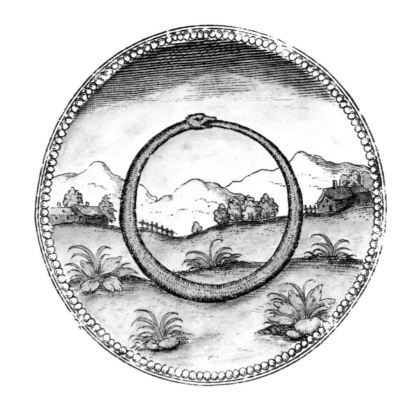

*If we see leaf, flower, and fruit
within the bud, this means that
we are seeing with the eyes of our
imagination.*
—Bachelard

Essences are volatile aromatic compounds of scent molecules that quickly become airborne vapors and reach our noses. You are already, and often, in the presence of natural essences—they are what make the heavenly aromas in fresh herbs and spices, citrus peel, vanilla bean. If you drag your fingernail along the skin of a lemon, it is the essence in the rind that transfers to your fingernail. Essences are where the fragrances live in plants; they can be extracted by various means, from hot steam to cold compressed gases. In fact, good-quality essences have an aroma and flavor whose intensity exceeds that available in the plant material itself. In concentrated liquid form, they are eminently suitable for creating fragrances and flavors.

The interior world of plants manifests itself in these essences. They come from every part of the plant: wood and bark (sandalwood, cinnamon), resin (frankincense, myrrh), root (ginger, vetiver), flower (rose, ylang ylang), leaf (basil, tarragon), seed (cumin, coriander), and rind (lemon, grapefruit).

Natural essences come in various types depending on their method of extraction:

essential oils,
CO$_2$ extracts,
absolutes,
and isolates.

ESSENTIAL OILS are the largest category of fragrance materials and the most widely available, thanks to the tremendous popularity of aromatherapy, which uses the essences for their therapeutic aromatic benefits. Plant materials are put through a process of distillation with water or steam. Many substances whose boiling points are far higher than that of water are volatilized out of the plant materials, and upon cooling they separate from the watery distillate and can be preserved in a relatively pure condition.

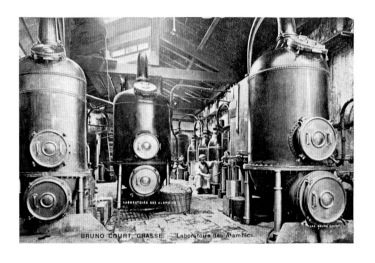

BRUNO COURT, GRASSE. Laboratoire des Alambics.

ABOVE
Laboratory of alembics used for distillation

RIGHT
The distillation of essential oils

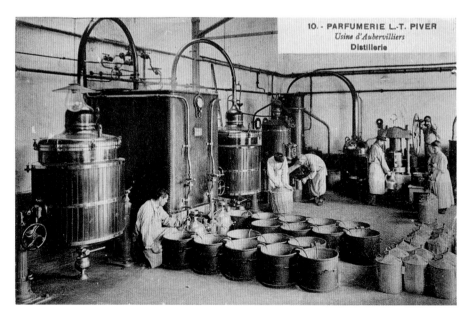

10.- PARFUMERIE L.-T. PIVER
Usine d'Aubervilliers
Distillerie

ABSOLUTES are created from materials too fragile for steam distillation—mostly flowers and spices, whose natural perfume molecules would decompose under the heat. The first process for capturing the tender aroma molecules from flowers was enfleurage, in which racks of petals rendered their fragrance into a fatty pomade, from which a powerfully scented oil was derived. Nowadays, natural flower oils are separated from fresh flowers by solvent extraction. The flowers are placed on racks in a hermetically sealed container. A liquid solvent, usually hexane, is circulated over the plant materials to dissolve the essential oils and yield an absolute. These highly concentrated liquid essences are much longer lasting than essential oils and have an unequaled intensity and fineness to their aroma. They are the most expensive perfumery ingredients.

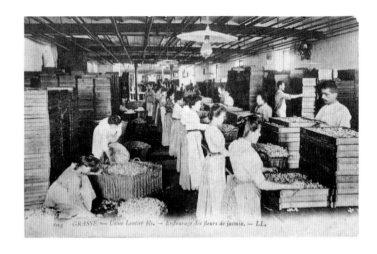

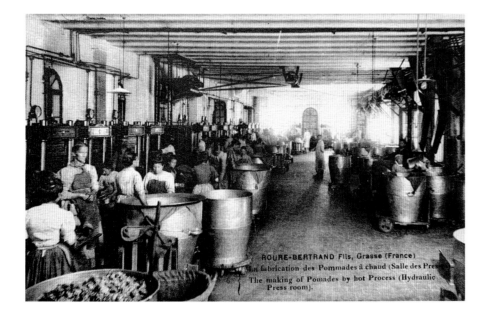

ABOVE
Enfleurage of jasmine

LEFT
Part of the enfleurage process: making floral pomades

C O₂ EXTRACTS use pressurized carbon dioxide (CO_2) as a solvent to extract the essential oil along with other substances. This can be done at lower temperatures than with water-based distillation. Thanks to the mild temperature range, CO_2-extracted oils remain closest in constitution to the oils in the plant itself.

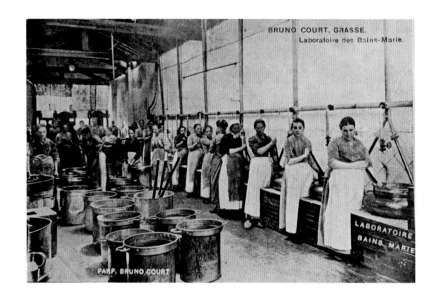

LEFT
Extracting essences at the Laboratoire des Bains-Marie

BELOW
Bottling essences

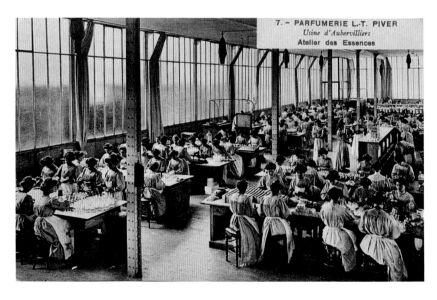

NATURAL ISOLATES are essences that are further processed to yield a simpler aroma. An essential oil is a cocktail, invented by nature, of different kinds of aroma molecules: major, minor, and trace constituents. A natural isolate is one of those aromatic components separated from the others, much as an egg yolk can be separated from the whole egg to be used in a recipe. The process is imperfect, and the resultant natural isolate is slightly contaminated, in the nicest possible way: it always includes trace amounts of other aroma molecules from the source essential oil. Natural isolates of the same aroma molecule therefore smell different depending on the essential oil source. Synthetic aroma molecules, however, are pure, and their aroma is less rounded and less complex than that of their natural counterparts. The trace aroma molecules make, for example, natural linalool isolated from ho wood warmer and more dimensional than synthetic linalool.

Among the first natural isolates were coumarin from tonka beans in 1868, vanillin from vanilla in 1874, and phenyl ethyl alcohol from rose in 1876. The isolation of single aroma molecules from natural sources played a decisive role in ushering in the use of synthetics in perfumery. Very soon after their discovery, natural isolates fell out of use in commercial perfumery, displaced by cheaper synthetic versions. Authentic natural isolates are filled with nuance and character, and are still used in artisanal natural perfumery to great effect.

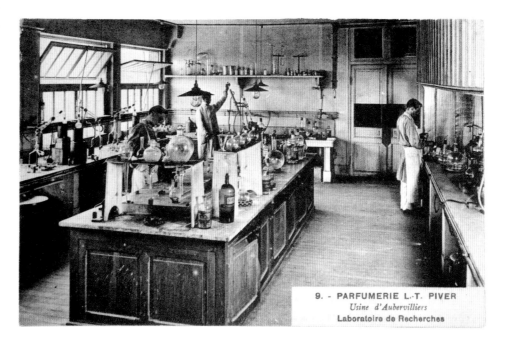

A perfume laboratory

9. - PARFUMERIE L.-T. PIVER
Usine d'Aubervilliers
Laboratoire de Recherches

Deconstructing an Essence

Like all natural essences, Turkish rose absolute is made up of hundreds of different aroma molecules or isolates. The five major rose isolates that occur in different proportions in all roses are

citronellol,
damascenone,
geraniol,
linalool, and
phenyl ethyl alcohol.

Constructing a Perfume

The essences that compose a perfume are called notes, and the notes are blended into chords, as in music.

The TOP CHORD creates the perfume's first impression. The top chord of my Boheme Confection perfume is composed of the following essences: methyl anthranilate, vanillin, sarsparilla, and bitter almond.

The MIDDLE CHORD forms the perfume's heart. The middle chord of Boheme Confection is composed of chocolate, pink lotus, and strawberry.

The BASE CHORD defines the perfume's lasting character. The base chord of Boheme Confection is composed of Peru balsam, benzoin, patchouli, and maltol.

Together the three chords create a harmonious whole that evolves as you wear it.

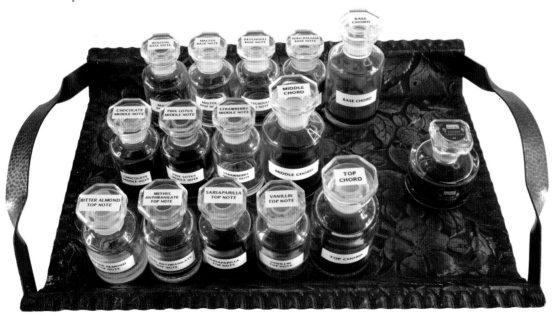

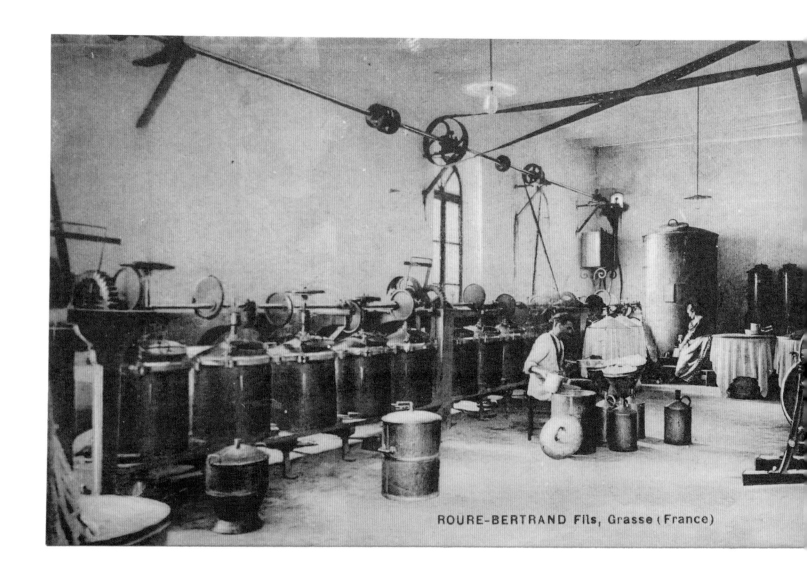

ROURE-BERTRAND Fils, Grasse (France)

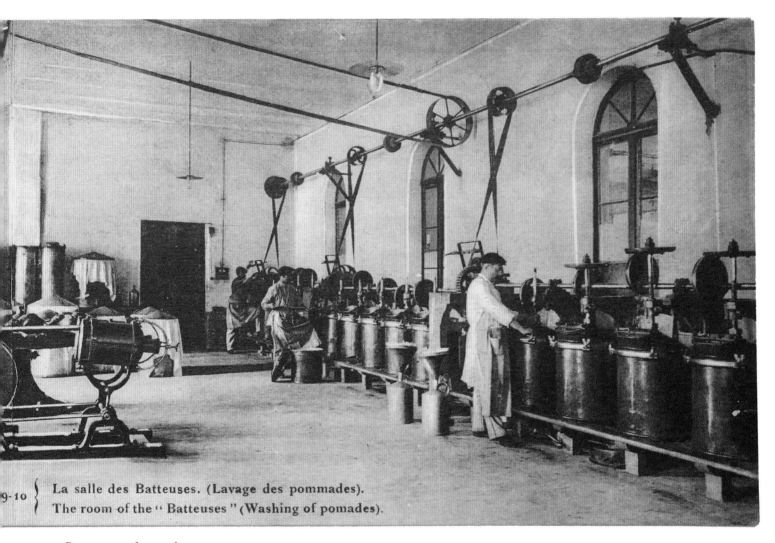

La salle des Batteuses. (Lavage des pommades).
The room of the " Batteuses " (Washing of pomades).

Panorama of pomades

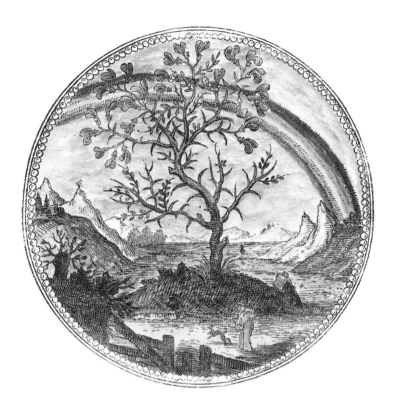

3
Perfume Organ

A perfume "organ" is dozens to hundreds of bottles filled with different aromatic botanical essences. It's called an organ because the essence bottles are arranged on shallow tiered shelves that look like a musical organ, and the essences are referred to as "notes" when a perfumer is composing a perfume.

The organ contains both familiar and unfamiliar essences. When you encounter aromas that you think you already know—chocolate, coffee, basil—you may find them beautiful, but the logical part of our brain tends to jump in to find words that match up to the experience: "That smells like basil." This rush to label tends to close a door to reverie, cutting off the imagination.

Unusual aromas—choya, mitti, ambrettolide, poplar buds—put a more expansive process in motion. Unfamiliar, unplaceable, unknown, and uncategorizable, they immerse us in our sensual response—the crucial first step in experiencing a scent. They open the door to funky and strange impressions, and then to the associations that are called up. This kind of raw encounter with beauty, vibrancy, and aliveness returns us to our bodies in the present moment.

You don't just smell an aroma; you fall into it. Then sensations and images arise, and you don't know whether you are dreaming or remembering. The present smell recalls an absent image. A smell is an integrating force—it draws together diverse impressions from memory and daydreams. When you actively participate in experiencing an aroma, you feel an inner movement and release. Mint is warmth and freshness, moss is humid softness, cumin is sweaty and earthy.

Scent families are a convenient way to keep track of the vast and diverse array of natural essences. Thinking of them in groups makes it easier to compare and contrast them and observe their individual character more closely. The greatest understanding of an aroma comes through recognizing minute differences between essences that smell similar, but not the same. For this reason I have grouped essences from the perfume organ in chapters of simple fragrance families as a starting point for thinking about them:

- Flowers *(page 27)*
- Woods *(page 61)*
- Leaves and grasses *(page 83)*
- Resins *(page 113)*
- Spices *(page 135)*
- Citruses *(page 167)*
- Gourmand *(page 197)*
- Herbs *(page 217)*
- Isolates *(page 238)*

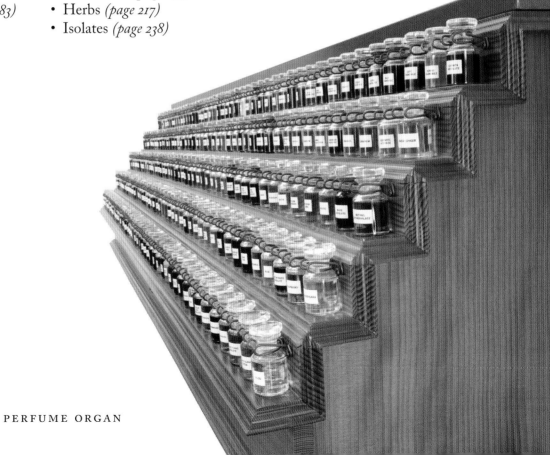

PERFUME ORGAN

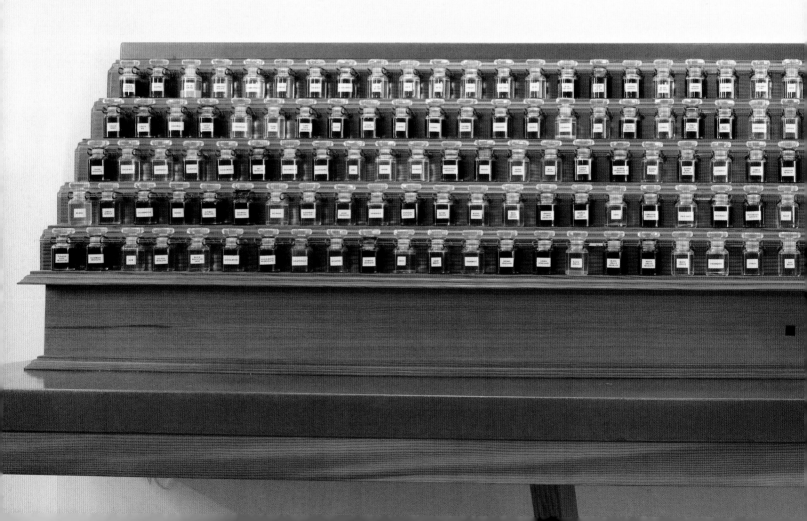

The perfume organ in the Aftel Archive. The artwork hanging above it is inscribed to Mandy Aftel, "the muse of the laboratory," by Leonard Cohen.

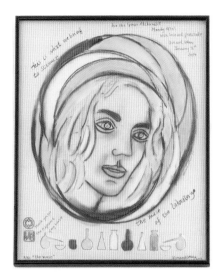

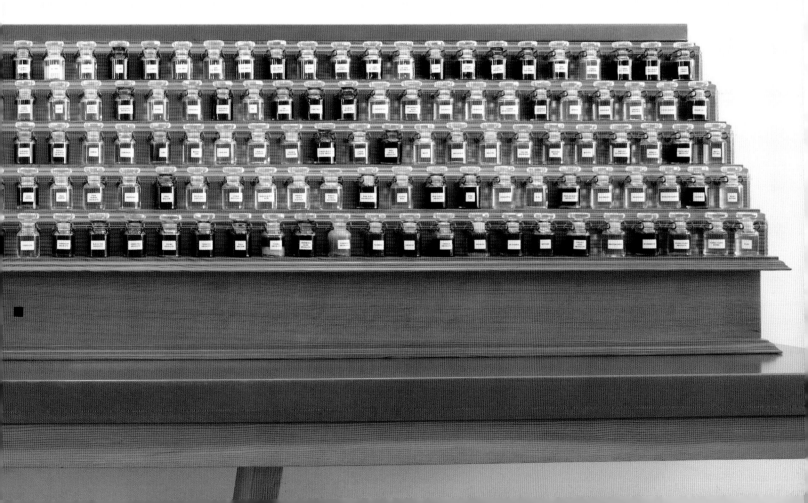

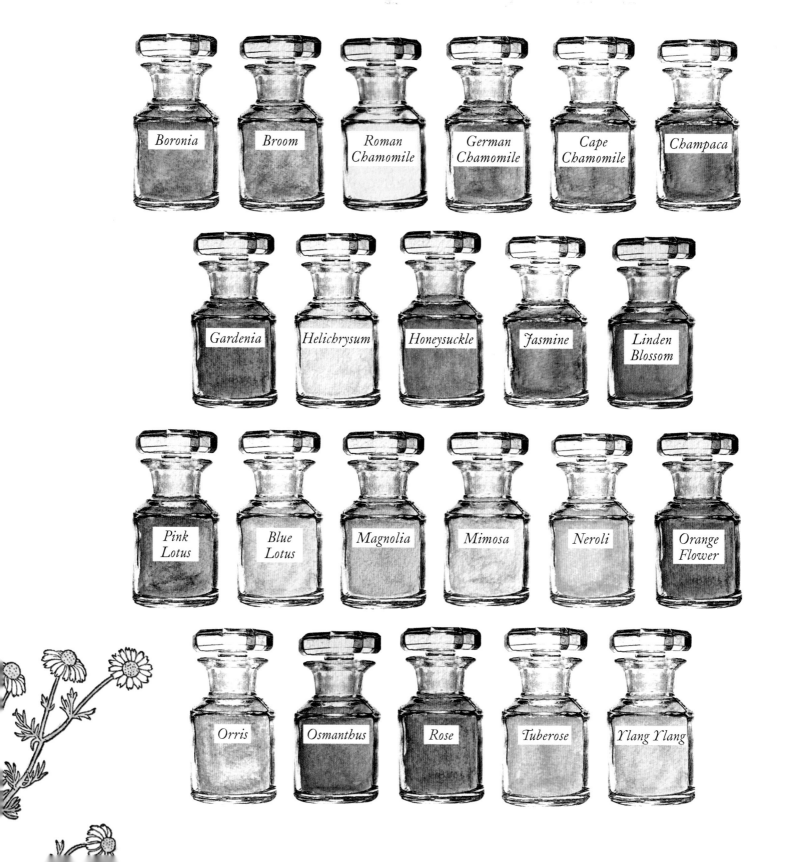

4
The Flower Family

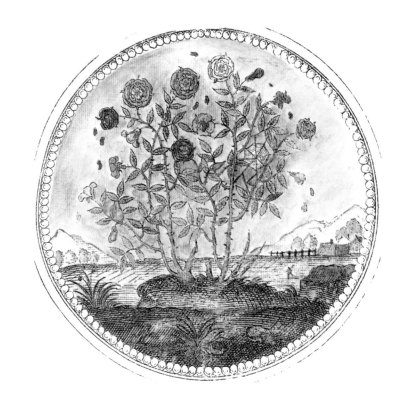

The intensity of interior beauty
condenses the beauties of an entire
universe. . . . The whole summer
is in a flower; the rose brims over
with inner space.
    —Bachelard

Flowers have always been used as tokens of love, and their gorgeous aromas are the fundamental building blocks of perfume. It can be difficult to collect flowers in amounts sufficient to extract their essence. The floral essences, as a group, are the costliest botanicals to create perfumes with. The incredibly complex floral aromas that nature puts together cannot be replicated synthetically. Often one iconic aroma predominates, but with it are associated traces of closely related molecules that shade and soften the predominant scent.

The creation of even a single flower feels miraculous: that a plant makes a flower, from the tiniest bud to the final bloom, is like a plant making a painting. A bud in its smallness contains the hugeness of the blossom to come; the fruit hides within the bud—and reveals its secret presence in the fruity facets that all floral aromas include. In fact, nature has built no flower scents around a single note—each is a bouquet, a complex work of art. Each contains a world in a single drop. Smelling a floral essence is like being around a flower that never wilts or dies—a flower with superpowers.

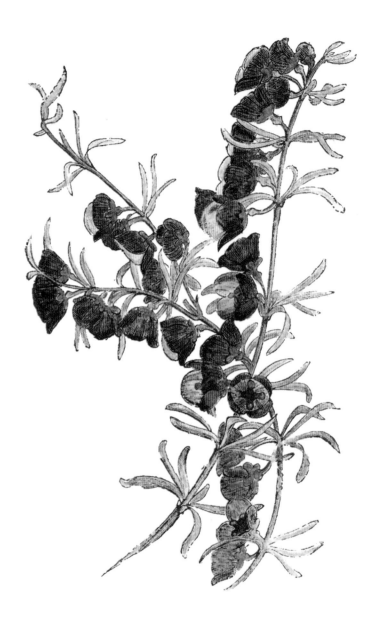

Boronia

Boronia megastigma

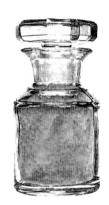

An ornamental bush with a delightful scent, graceful form, and flowers with unusual coloration. Boronia was not available in classical European perfumes. Grown and produced in Tasmania, it is one of the few perfume ingredients that is indigenous to a particular area, representative of that terroir, and not found anywhere else.

Boronia is a delicate, very expensive floral that smells like a combination of raspberry, apricot, and freesia. Boronia contains two ionones—alpha and beta—the aroma molecules that smell like violets. It is a very unusual aroma with a sheer texture, providing the perfumer novel tonalities to work with.

Available as an absolute

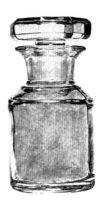

Broom

Spartium junceum

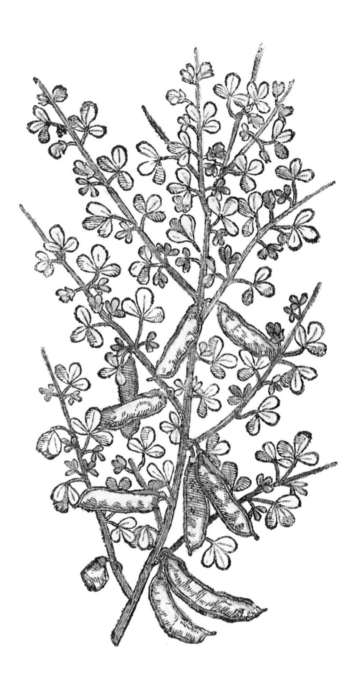

This plant is called "broom" because its twigs are made into brooms. Its fragrant, yellow-golden flowers grow wild, broadcasting a rich and intensely sweet aroma in the sunlight. The flowers must be worked with quickly, as their aroma deteriorates once they are cut.

Broom offers an uncanny mixture of aromas both rich and delicate: it has an almost edible aroma of wild dark-colored honey and the flowers it comes from, along with raisins and hay.

Available as an absolute

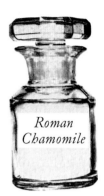

Roman Chamomile

Chamo-
mile

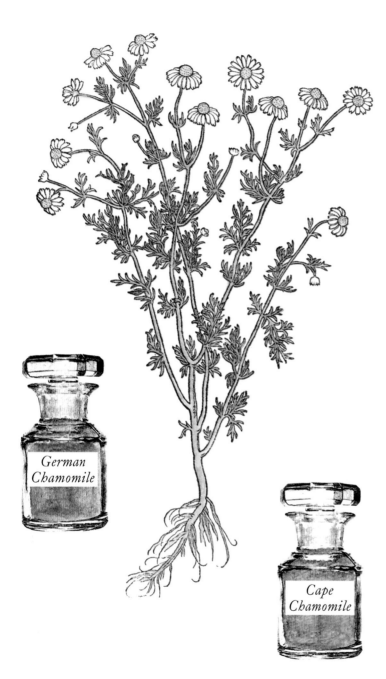

German Chamomile

Cape Chamomile

Being stepped on is beneficial to chamomile, which is one of the reasons why it is often planted in walkways. When the plant is walked on, the strong apple fragrance will reveal its presence even before it is seen.

Roman chamomile (*Anthemis nobilis* or *Chamaemelum nobile*), with its scent of green apples, was made famous as a tea by Peter Rabbit. The flowers are used for their anti-inflammatory and sedative capacities.

The deep blue essential oil distilled from German chamomile (*Matricaria recutita* or *Matricaria chamomilla*) has a strong bitter aroma but is incredibly therapeutic. Its blue color is due to chamazulene, a chemical compound derived only from chamomile and a few other plants.

Cape chamomile *(Eriocephalus punctulatus)*, a lesser-known variety of the plant, yields my favorite of the chamomile essential oils, with its hypnotic light green-blue color and a boozy fruity, floral aroma. All three of the chamomiles are known to be very calming.

Available as essential oils

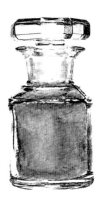

Champaca

Michelia champaca
(or *Magnolia champaca*)

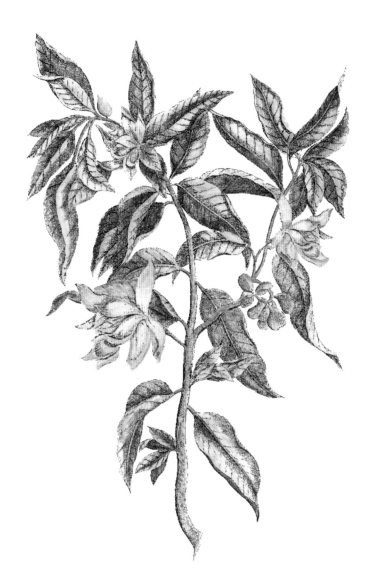

Champaca, a member of the magnolia family, has a smooth, velvety, heady floral aroma. When the tree blooms—once in the monsoon season and once more in the spring—it is covered in golden flowers exuding a heavy, diffusive fragrance. Champaca absolute has more than 240 fragrance molecules in its complex aroma profile, including indole (jasmine), ionones (violet), and methyl anthranilate (orange blossom). Indole adds an animalic facet to the spicy floral aroma, which is almost edible—reminiscent of a deeply roasted rare oolong tea. It is heavy yet refreshing, soothing yet disturbing: an aromatic reconciliation of opposites.

Although both are derived from trees of the magnolia family, champaca absolute is not to be confused with magnolia essential oil. (See page 39.)

Available as an absolute

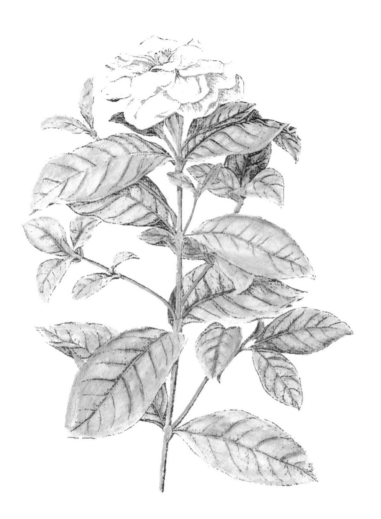

Gardenia

Gardenia taitensis

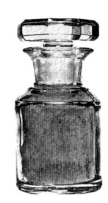

Intense, rich, creamy, and sweet, the Tahitian gardenia, also known as tiaré, is the gold standard of voluptuousness. Named for Dr. Alexander Garden, an eighteenth-century Scottish naturalist, gardenia is the symbol of Tahiti specifically and Polynesia in general. People there link the blossoms together in strands that they wear on their bodies for special occasions, the flowers being even more fragrant in the damp night air. The heady, creamy tropical aroma is heavy with notes of mango, guava, and passion fruit.

Available, but rarely found, as an absolute

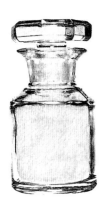

Helichry-sum

Helichrysum italicum (or *Helichrysum angustifolium*)

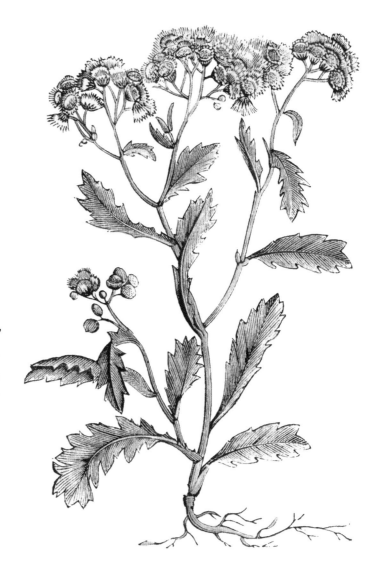

Helichrysum means "golden sun": *helios* is Greek for "sun" and *chrysos* is Greek for "gold," referring to the plant's small golden flowers. The essential oil, steam distilled from the flower, has a warm, sweet, herbaceous aroma with honey and tea facets. Also beautifully called "everlasting" and "immortelle," it has a delicate and diffusive aroma that is both calming and soothing.

Available as an essential oil and an absolute

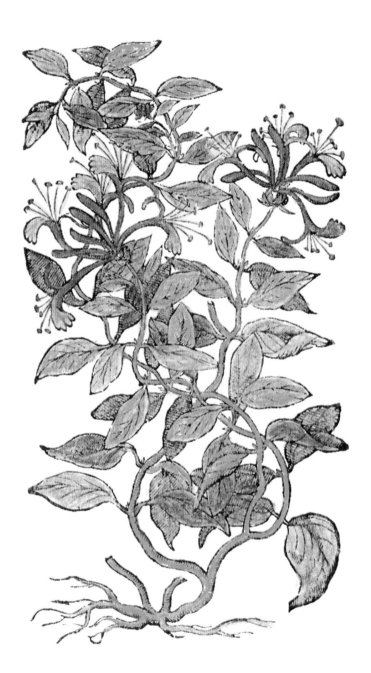

Honey-suckle

Lonicera fragrantissima

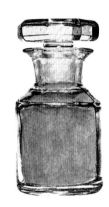

Honeysuckle used to be called "woodbine," because it binds itself to every tree and shrub growing nearby. The plant is pollinated by sphinx moths that behave like hummingbirds—just hovering in front of the flowers. The flowers are almost odorless during the day but become very fragrant and diffusive in the evening. Honeysuckle's beautiful fruity, floral aroma is balanced with facets of eugenol (clove) and vanillin (vanilla), giving it sweet undertones like gardenia. It doesn't have the heaviness of some florals, but a brighter springtime aroma.

Available as an extremely rare absolute

Woodbine, or Honey-Suckles

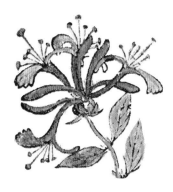

It is a plant so common, that every one that hath eyes knows it, and he that hath none, cannot read a description, if I should write it.

[Time.] They flower in June, and the fruit is ripe in August.

[Government and Virtues] Doctor Tradition, that grand introducer of errors, that hater of truth, lover of folly, and that mortal foe to Doctor Reason, hath taught the common people to use the leaves or flowers of this plant in mouth-water, and by long continuance of time, that so grounded it in the brains of the vulgar, that you cannot beat it out with a beetle; All mouth-waters ought to be cooling and drying, but honey-suckles are cleansing, consuming and digesting, and therefore no way fit for inflammations; thus Dr. Reason. Again if you please we will leave Dr. Reason awhile, and come to Dr. Experience, a learned gentleman, and his brother; take a leaf and chew it in your mouth, and you will quickly find it likelier to cause a sore mouth and throat than cure it. Well then, if it be not good for this, what is it good for? It is good for something, for God and nature made nothing in vain. It is an herb of Mercury, and appropriated to the lungs; the Celestial Crab claims dominion over it, neither is it a foe to the Lion; if the lungs be afflicted by Jupiter, this is your cure: it is fitting a conserve made of the flowers of it were kept in every gentlewoman's house; I know no better cure for asthma than this; Besides, it takes away the evil of the spleen, provokes urine, procures speedy delivery of women in travail, helps cramps, convulsions, and palsies, and whatsoever griefs come of cold or stopping; if you please to make use of it as an ointment, it will clear your skin of morphew, freckles, and sun burnings, or whatever else discolours it, and then the maids will love it. Authors say, the flowers are of more effect than the leaves and that is true; But they say the seeds are least effectual of all. But Dr. Reason told me, that there was a vital spirit in every seed to beget its like; and Dr. Experience told me, that there was a greater heat in the seed than there was in any other part of the plant; And withal, that heat was the mother of action, and then judge if old Dr. Tradition (who may well be honored for his age, but not for his goodness) hath not so poisoned the world with errors before I was born, that it was never well in its wits since, and there is great fear it will die mad.

—Culpepper, *The English Physician*, 1807 edition, pp. 277–78

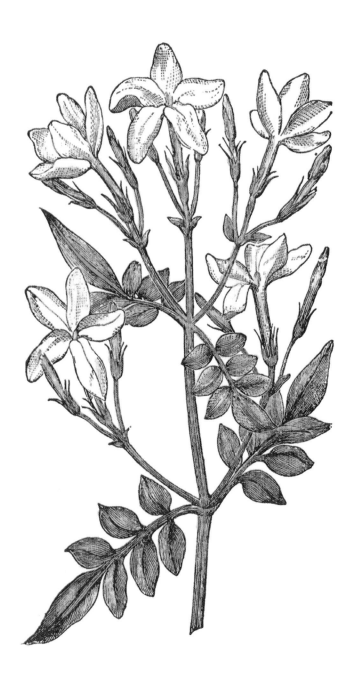

Jasmine

Jasminum grandiflorum
and *Jasminum sambac*

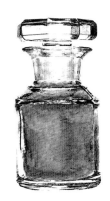

Jasmine is the aromatic equivalent of the king of beasts. There is no essence that comes close to it—and synthetics can't replicate it! Jasmine's aroma is narcotic and heady, lightened by fruit-scented molecules and balsamic notes. Two species of jasmine are used in creating perfume: *grandiflorum*, which is sweet, floral, rich; and *sambac*, which is spicy and less sweet or floral, and therefore considered more "masculine."

The sweet, heavy, diffusive, sensuous scent of jasmine is immediately familiar to anyone in Northern California who has taken a walk outdoors at night. Jasmine embodies the yin-yang duality—at once sultry and dirty, even fecal—that makes scent a catalyst for sexual attraction. Its narcotic lushness reminds us that beauty needs ugliness to exist at all. Pure gorgeousness would be bland and insipid without the foil of its counterpart. An important aroma molecule in jasmine is indole, which is also in feces! This lends jasmine its bipolar ability to be drop-dead gorgeous and slightly putrid at the same time. Without that *jolie laide* aspect of beauty, it would be simpler but less compelling. Jasmine flowers continue to develop and emit their natural perfume even after being detached from the plant.

Available as absolutes

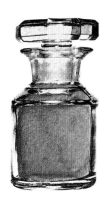

Linden Blossom

Tilia cordata
(or *Tilia ×europaea*)

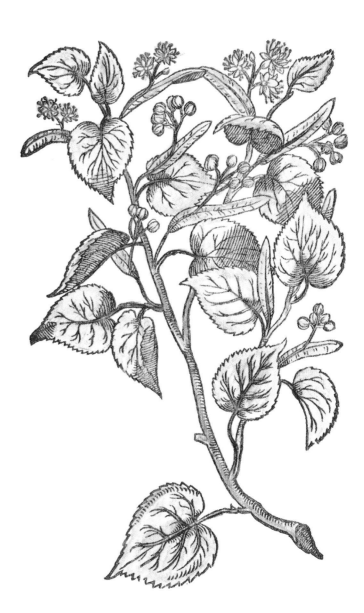

Linden has heart-shaped leaves and greenish yellow flowers that give off a honeyed floral scent of lilies and lilacs with touches of rose and lime. Linden blossoms are only faintly scented during the day, but in the night air, they diffuse their delightfully sweet floral aroma. Linden essence has a delicate warm, fruity, hay-like floral aroma.

Available as an absolute and a CO_2

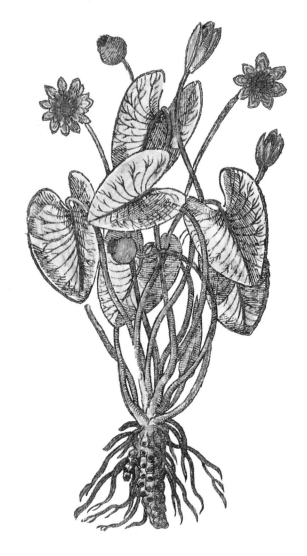

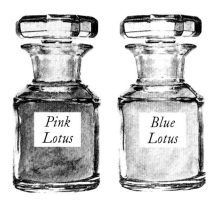

Lotus

The lotuses are dramatic aquatic plants with their roots in the mud at the bottom of the water, and their flowers and leaves on the water's surface.

Pink lotus (*Nelumbo nucifera*), easier to find and less expensive than blue, has a rich, dense, spicy, full-bodied floral aroma.

Blue lotus (*Nymphaea caerulea*) is luminous, honeyed, transcendent, and mesmerizing. It was the most important scented plant in ancient Egypt from the Twelfth Dynasty on, and played a prominent role in Egyptian mythology and religion. It also has a long-standing association with Buddhism. Blue lotus is rumored to have a psychotropic effect, and may have been the narcotic plant consumed by the Lotus Eaters in Homer's *Odyssey*.

Available as absolutes

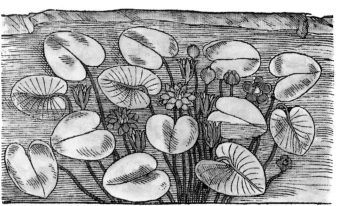

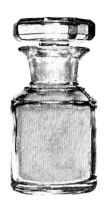

Magnolia

Michelia ×alba
(or *Magnolia ×alba*)

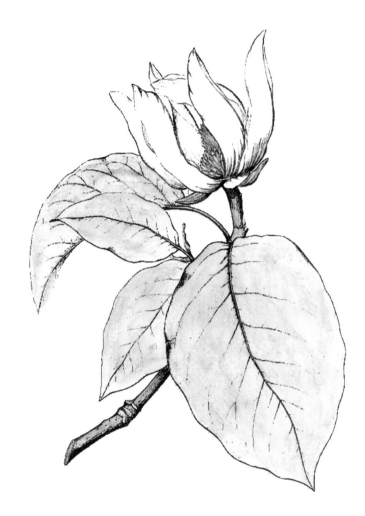

Michelia *alba*'s essential oil, called magnolia essential oil, has a fresh, sweet, fruity floral aroma, like a marriage of geranium and ylang ylang. There is some confusion between magnolia essential oil (*Michelia alba*) and champaca absolute (*Michelia champaca*), since their names are similar and both are in the magnolia family. It is from *Michelia champaca* that we get the luscious, heavy and deeply floral champaca absolute. (See page 31.) And, to confuse things even more, neither of them is the magnolia that is grown in the United States, which is *Magnolia grandiflora*.

Available as an essential oil

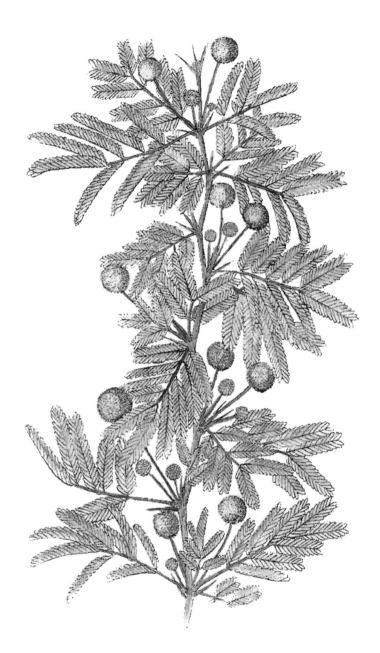

Mimosa

Acacia farnesiana
(or *Vachellia farnesiana*)

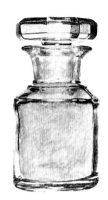

Mimosa looks like a yellow puffball, because the stamens of the flower are longer than the petals. Its aroma is powdery, sweet, soft, and flat, with low odor intensity. Although it's very sweet, it's a light sweetness, not a full-bodied honey sweetness. Mimosa is a good floral supporting character, blending well and smoothing other essences. It is one of the most inexpensive florals.

Available as an absolute

Neroli & Orange Flower

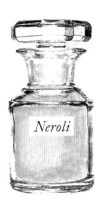

Citrus ×aurantium

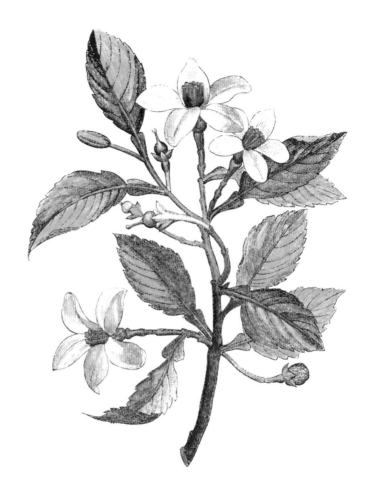

Orange flower makes you rethink the smell of orange entirely. The bitter orange tree is a perfume industry all unto itself, yielding four different essences: one from the fruit (bitter orange essential oil), one from the leaves and twigs (petitgrain essential oil), and two from the flowers (neroli essential oil and orange flower absolute).

Marie Anna de la Tremoille, princess of Nerola (1670–1722), loved the fragrance of orange flowers and was the first to have it distilled for perfuming her gloves and her bath. The light and refreshing neroli essential oil was named after her.

Orange flower absolute is the most expensive, rarest, and most complex of all the bitter orange aromas. Perfumers favor bitter orange over sweet orange because the sweetness gets in the way of the orange aroma. Once orange is blended with bitterness, the aroma becomes a suave and restrained reconciliation of opposites—citrus and floral, bright and heady, heavy and delicate. Orange flower also has a dirty facet due to the presence of the aroma molecule indole.

Available as a cool, elegant, intense, suave absolute and as neroli, a lighter and more citrusy essential oil

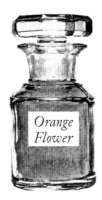

Odors of orange-flowers, and spice,
Reached them from time to time,
Like airs that breathe from Paradise
Upon a world of crime.

—Longfellow

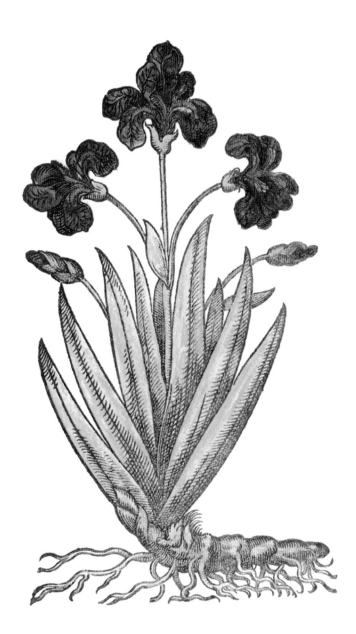

Orris

Iris ×germanica

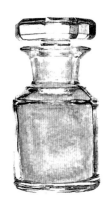

In ancient Greece and Rome, orris root was used as both a perfume and as a medicine, back when there was no distinction between the two. *Iris ×germanica* is known in India by its Persian name, *bikh-i-banafshah*, which means "violet root." Orris root, mixed with anise, was used as a perfume for linens as early as 1480.

Fresh orris root is practically odorless. The characteristic odor, which resembles violets, develops during the drying process and is probably due to fermentation. Before they can be used, the roots have to be stored for three years to bring out the full powdery-soft violet aroma. When steam distilled, the extract solidifies into violet-scented orris "butter."

Available as orris butter

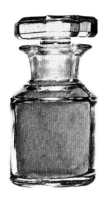

Osmanthus

Osmanthus fragrans

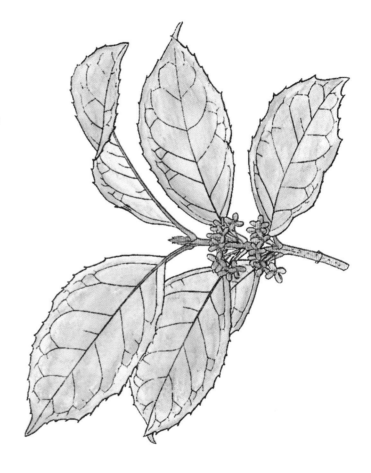

Osmanthus, an evergreen bush from the olive family, blooms year-round and is considered the scent of China. Much like jasmine, the flowers have been used in China to enhance the finest green and black teas. The absolute has a remarkable 370 constituents, including beta ionone and damascenone, which are also present in tea leaves. Osmanthus is a very complicated floral essence to work with—there's a unique balance between the different facets of its aroma: the rich floral notes, the dried fruit notes, and the putrid ones. Think ripe apricots and humidity.

Available as an absolute

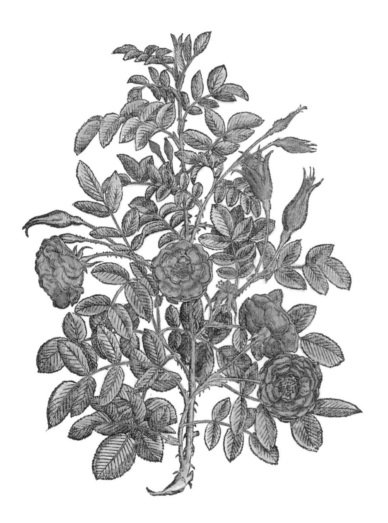

Rose

Rosa ×damascena
and *Rosa ×centifolia*

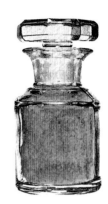

Prized around the world for its gorgeous, iconic look and aroma, the rose's many origin myths include springing from the blood of Venus or Adonis, or the sweat of Muhammad. The process of extracting rose essential oil was discovered in 1574.

Some consider the rose emblematic of joy, and others of silence. At feasts, when conversations were to be held in secret, a rose would be suspended above the table, hence the term "sub rosa." Long ago men of rank had their mattresses filled with dried rose petals.

Rose notes may vary considerably one from another, depending on where the rose was grown and how its essence was extracted. The range always includes rosy, with possible notes of honey or butter or spice or fruit or some ingenious combination. The texture is soft and round and rich.

Rose essence can be distilled as an essential oil called an otto, or solvent-extracted to yield an absolute. Rose otto is light colored and its aroma is sheerer and lighter, whereas rose absolute is richer in color (deep

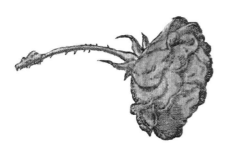

red) and aroma. Among rose essences there is infinite variation from the presence of more than 300 aroma compounds. The best rose essences are multilayered, rich, and full of possibilities. Although rose essence contains 0.1% damascenone (plummy, fruity) and 33% citronellol (light rosy), the damascenone has a greater impact on the aroma.

Rose is welcome in any perfume, as there are very few essences that it doesn't get along with. When employed in a small amount, rose essence will just disappear into the background, smoothing down less harmonious essences that are sharp or difficult. When rose is used as a main essence, it enhances every other essence and contributes the unbelievably gorgeous smell of rose.

Around the world, rose essence has been used to flavor both sweet and savory dishes, and it was an important ingredient in early recipes for ginger ale.

Available as an essential oil and as an absolute

In further illustration of the capricious nature of the smell of rose, and the extraordinary complexity of its forms, it is stated that not only in the whole list of roses are there no two which develop precisely the same odour, but that in the same species, and even on the same plant, there are not found two flowers absolutely identical in odour—even yet further, that it is a well-known fact amongst rose growers that at different times in the day an individual flower will emit a different perfume.
—Sawyer, *Odorgraphia*, 1892

In Bulgaria the flowers grown for the distillation of the rose otto are gathered before they commence to open, and a little before sunrise. Were they gathered later in the day, when fully expanded by the heat, the perfume would be stronger, but not so sweet, and the resulting essence would be of less value.
—Sawyer, *Odorgraphia*, 1892

It has been noticed that previous to a storm, or atmospheric disturbance, the odour of the rose seems strangely increased; this may be by reason of the oxidizing influence of the ozone in the atmosphere, or it may be that our perceptive faculties are sharpened at such moments.
—Sawyer, *Odorgraphia*, 1892

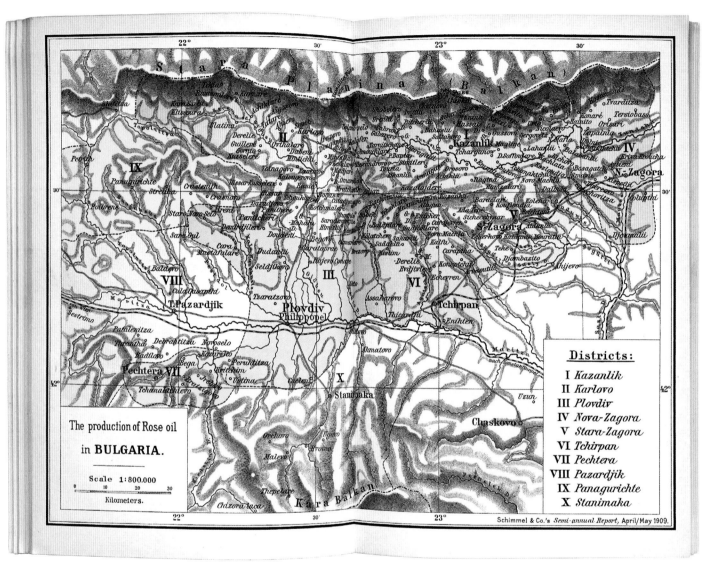

The production of Rose oil in **BULGARIA**.

Scale 1:800.000

0   10   20   30
Kilometers.

Districts:
I *Kazanlik*
II *Karlovo*
III *Plovdiv*
IV *Nova-Zagora*
V *Stara-Zagora*
VI *Tchirpan*
VII *Pechtera*
VIII *Pazardjik*
IX *Panagurichte*
X *Stanimaka*

Schimmel & Co.'s *Semi-annual Report*, April/May 1909.

Map of roses in Bulgaria, Schimmel & Co., 1909

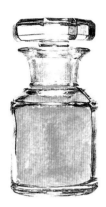

Tuberose

Polianthes tuberosa
(or *Agave amica*)

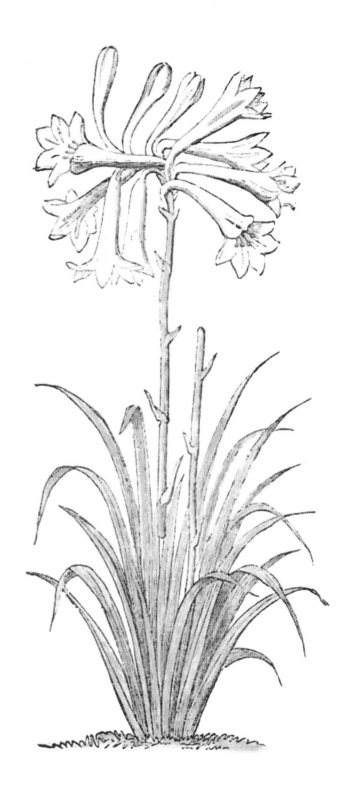

Tuberose is a symbol of voluptuousness: a single intoxicating stem smells like an entire flower garden. Not a tuber and not a rose, the upright growth stands tall like a row of soldiers. Heavy and overpowering, tuberose comes to life at night as its heady, sweet, sensuous odor intensifies. The flower continues to make perfume after it is picked. Tuberose was domesticated by pre-Columbian peoples in Mexico. It is an intense mixture of aromas: a narcotic floral, and earthy wild mushrooms balanced with creamy lactones.

Available as an absolute

A wonderful bouquet, which has been compared with the perfume of a well-stocked flower garden at evening close. In the east, these white tubular flowers emit a most powerful odor, which increases after sunset.
—Poucher, *Perfumes and Cosmetics*, 1923

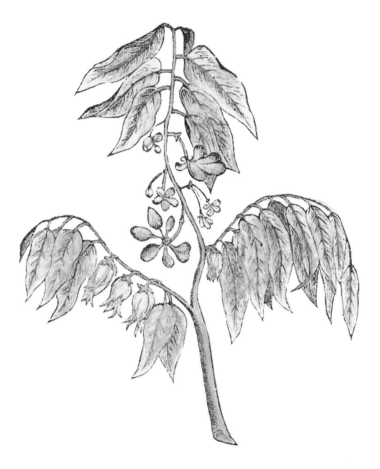

Ylang Ylang

Cananga odorata

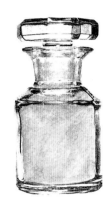

As with olive oil, there are first, second, and third renderings of ylang ylang oil, with the first labeled as "extra," connoting the highest grade. The flowers start out green and, in a few days, turn yellow and develop a spicy, creamy floral note. Ylang ylang is unique in having a banana facet in its floral aroma—overripe bananas to be precise, the ones where the skin is all brown, the flesh is soft, and the sweetness oozes out to meet you. The fruitiness is balanced with a dollop of spicy cinnamon and nutmeg.

Available as an essential oil, concrete, and absolute. The concrete is my favorite.

5
Ambergris

*The origin of ambergris was for many years an unfathomable mystery. Found floating on the sea it gave no clew to the place or manner of its formation, and, from a supposed analogy to amber, took the name it still bears—*gray *amber. Within a comparatively recent period, however, it has been traced to the* Physeter macrocephalus, *or spermaceti whale. This mammal seems at times to suffer with a kind of indigestion, or torpidity of the stomach and intestines, the consequence of which is a deposit in those organs of the substance known as ambergris.*

—Snively, *Manufacture of Perfumes*, 1877

There is no substance in the world that embodies the idea of alchemy as ambergris does, a miracle of transformation that starts out soft, dense, jet black, and fecal, and ages in the ocean into a porous golden, gray, or white material with a gorgeous, almost unearthly scent.

The substance originates in the bowels of about one out of a hundred sperm whales, apparently caused by the irritation of cuttlefish beaks eaten by the whale. Expelled into the ocean, it may float upon the waves for decades, gradually transformed by sun and salt, before it is deposited on the beach, where from time to time it is discovered by the curious.

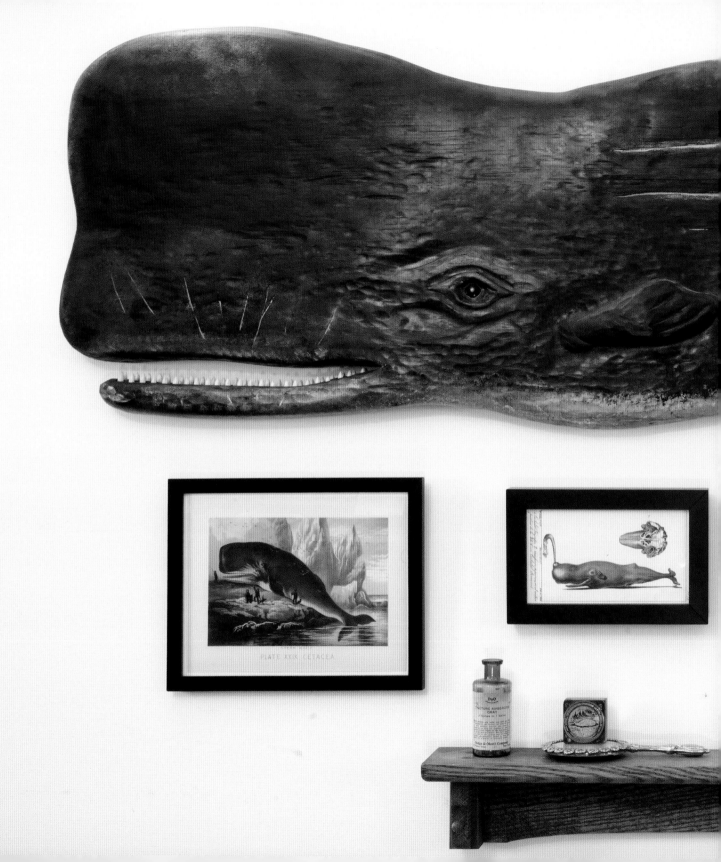

PLATE XXIX CETACEA

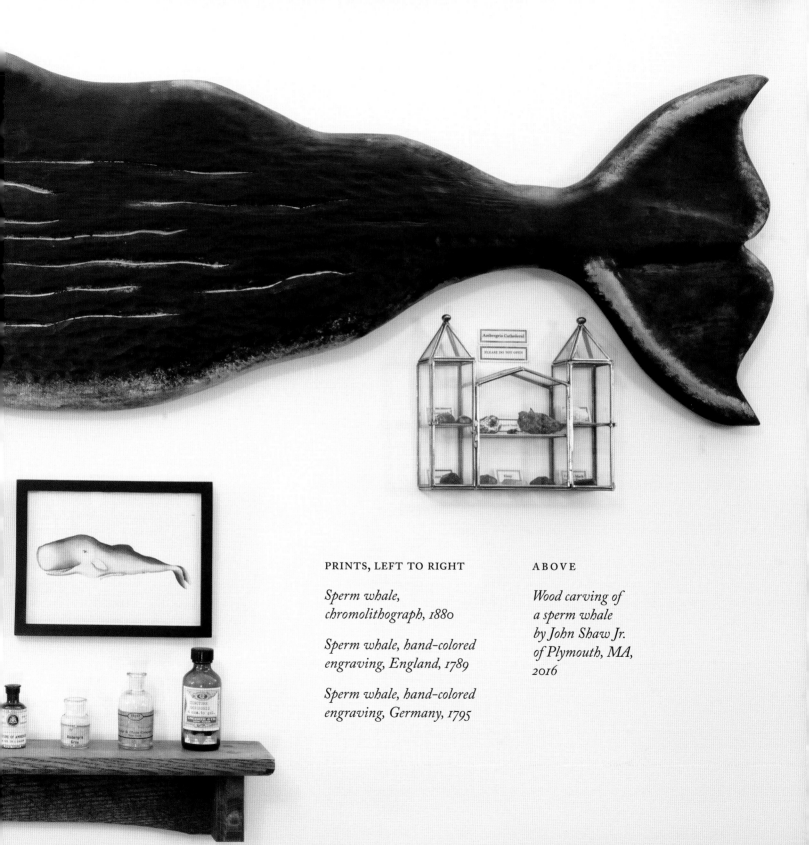

PRINTS, LEFT TO RIGHT

*Sperm whale,
chromolithograph, 1880*

*Sperm whale, hand-colored
engraving, England, 1789*

*Sperm whale, hand-colored
engraving, Germany, 1795*

ABOVE

*Wood carving of
a sperm whale
by John Shaw Jr.
of Plymouth, MA,
2016*

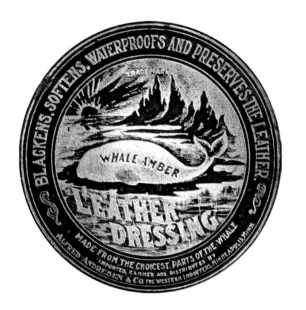

Stories about finding ambergris rival those of the discovery of the Maltese Falcon. A report from the 1930s claimed that some Hawaiian cowboys noticed masses of what they took to be sponge in the ocean and thought to use them to wipe down their ponies. Discovering that the material was not sponge, they took a sample to a local merchant, who identified it as ambergris. They hurried back to the spot where they had found it and managed to salvage enough to make them all financially independent for life.

The finest ambergris develops an incomparably lovely, sweet, musky odor that seems to combine perfume, the sea, and some primordial animal scent. Ambergris tincture has a warm and sweet sparkly, ambery scent.

BELOW LEFT
Century-old gray ambergris tincture bottle, Dodge and Olcott

BELOW RIGHT
Copper printing block, Whale Amber Leather Dressing, c. 1900. (See inset above left.)

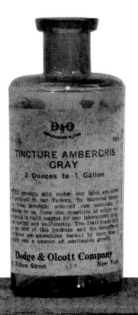

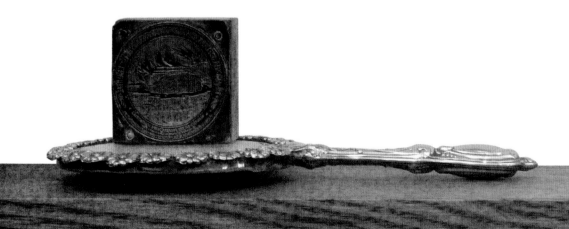

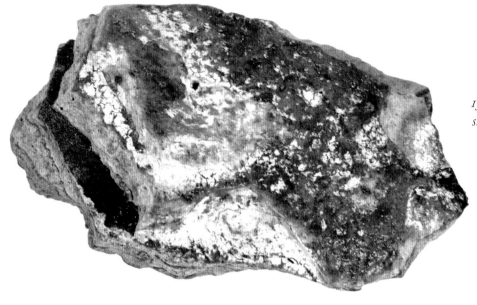

150-gram chunk of ambergis,
shown larger than actual size

BELOW
Century-old bottles, left to right:
Fritzsche Brothers ambergris tincture
Fritzsche Brothers gray ambergris tincture
Dodge and Olcott ambreine
Ungerer gray ambergris tincture

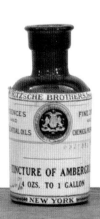
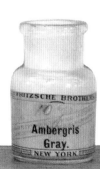
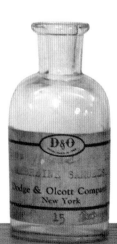
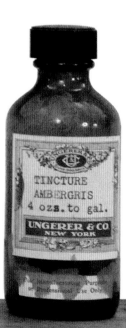

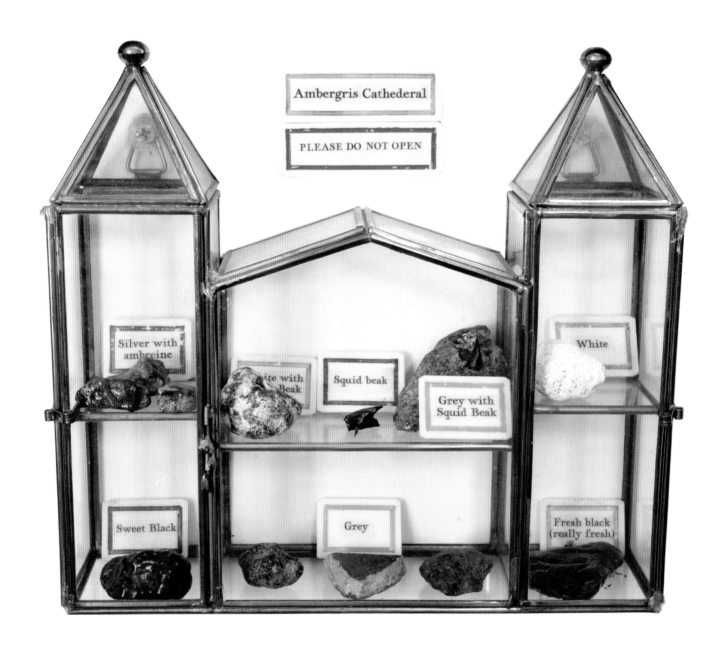

Ambergris cathedral. Specimens donated by
Adrienne Beuse of www.ambergris.co.nz.

6
Theatrum Botanicum

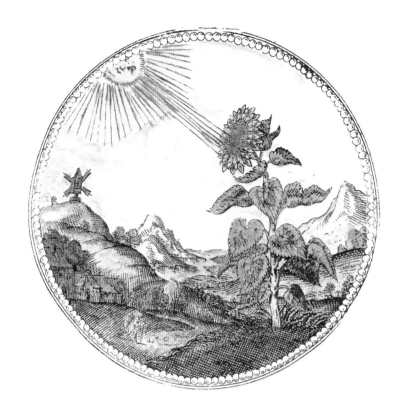

T*heatrum Botanicum* is the largest of the English herbals. The author, John Parkinson (1567–1650), was apothecary to King James I. He published his life's work, the massive *Theatrum Botanicum*, in 1640, when he was seventy-three years old! He was a member of the Grocers' Company, founded in 1345, the London trade guild that included pepperers and spicers as well as apothecaries. He was among the apothecaries who broke away in 1617 to found their own association, the Worshipful Society of Apothecaries. At that time apothecaries could practice medicine, and they relied on pharmacy books—which also included formulas for perfumes that they could sell in their shops.

Theatrum Botanicum, the "Theater of Plants," covers more than 4,000 plants and contains 2,700 woodcuts focusing on medicinal plants. The woodcuts are executed by several artists, and many are borrowed from an earlier herbal by Pietro Andrea Mattioli. The plants are inventively divided into seventeen "classes or tribes," mainly based on their medicinal qualities:

THEATRUM BO-
TANICVM:
THE
THEATER OF PLANTS.
OR,
AN HERBALL OF
A
LARGE EXTENT:

Containing therein a more ample and
exact Hiſtory and declaration of the Phyſicall Herbs
and Plants that are in other Authours, encreaſed by the acceſſe of
many hundreds of new, rare, and ſtrange Plants from all the parts of
the world, with ſundry Gummes, and other Phyſicall materials, than hath beene hitherto publiſhed by any before ; And
a moſt large demonſtration of their Natures and Vertues.

Shewing vvithall the many errors, differences, and
overſights of ſundry Authors that have formerly written of
them ; and a certaine confidence, or moſt probable con-
jecture of the true and genuine Herbes
and Plants.

Diſtributed into ſundry Claſſes or Tribes, for the
more eaſie knowledge of the many Herbes of one nature
and property, with the chiefe notes of Dr. Lobel, Dr. Bonham,
and others inſerted therein.

Collected by the many yeares travaile, induſtry, and experience in this
ſubject, by John Parkinſon Apothecary of London, and the
Kings Herbariſt.

And Publiſhed by the Kings Majeſtyes eſpeciall priviledge.

LONDON,
Printed by Tho. Cotes. 1640.

1. sweet-smelling plants
2. purging plants
3. venomous, sleepy, and hurtful plants and their counterpoisons
4. saxifrages or breakstone plants
5. vulnerary or wound herbs
6. cooling and succory-like herbs
7. hot and sharp biting plants
8. umbelliferous plants
9. thistles and thorny plants
10. ferns and capillary herbs
11. pulses
12. cereals
13. grasses, rushes, and reeds
14. marsh, water, and sea plants, and mosses and mushrooms
15. the unordered tribe
16. trees and shrubs
17. strange and outlandish plants

OPPOSITE
The title page of the Aftel Archive's copy of Theatrum Botanicum, *a first edition of 1640 published in London*

The book even includes the unicorn's horn, because it had been reported to be useful as a test for poisoned drinks!

Botany and medicine traveled together through the ages until the seventeenth century, when they parted ways: medical books no longer included anything about plants, and botanical books said little about the medicinal properties of plants. *Theatrum Botanicum* was a late example of the earlier type of book, called an "herbal," that had combined botany and medicine. Herbals contained botanical classifications, traditional plant lore, and notes on the plants' medicinal properties, including many "simples," or herbal remedies based on a single plant. Herbals also contain some of the earliest drawings of plants, which were a highly valued aid to identification. Many of the old illustrations were colored by hand or, if left black and white, were intended to be colored later. Illustrated herbals had a continuous history from the ancient Greeks to the end of the Middle Ages, alongside a similar type of book about animals, known as a "bestiary."

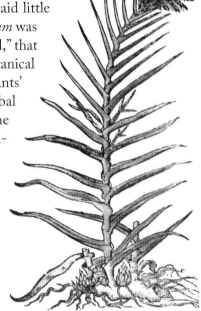

A spread from the
Aftel Archive's copy of
Theatrum Botanicum

11. 12. *Ranunculus Illyricuus major & minor.*
The greater & lesser *Slavonian* Crowfoote.

13. *Ranunculus Lusitanicus autumnalis.*
The Portugall Crowfoote.

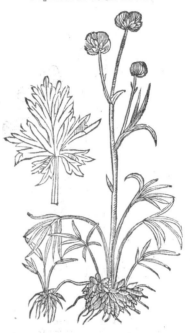

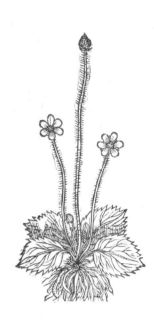

pled or swolne leaues, like as it were blisters upon them, and bearing the flower with eight or ten leaues, some-times as if it were double, whereof he giueth a figure, but the seede will beare such like plants, as he setteth forth the other to be, and therefore giueth no other mention or description thereof.

14. *Ranunculus autumnalis flore multiplici.* Double flowred Autumne Crowfoote.
This is so like the last in the manner of the growing and flowring, that onely the double yellow flowers make the difference.

15. *Ranunculus grumosa radice Bononiensis.* Meddow Crowfoote of *Bononia* with kernelly rootes.
This Crowfoote hath a roote made of many small long and round white kernels, or graines set close together, with diuerse long fibres at them, from whence rise up somewhat round leaues, but deepely cut in on the edges, into three parts, somewhat like unto those of the round rooted Crowfoote, sustained by long foote stalkes, and somewhat hayrie : from among which rise up the stalkes, that are hayrie also, and about a foote high, having leaues set thereon at two seuerall distances, much more cut in and jagged than those below, not divided into many branches, whose flowers at the tops of them are yellow, like unto other field Crowfeete : the small head of rough seede that followeth, is sharpe pointed, and shorter than others.

16. *Ranunculus Geranii tuberosi folio.* Iagged Field Crowfeete of *Padoa.*
The rootes of this Crowfeete consist of long whitish strings, sending forth many darke greene smooth leaues, very much jagged or cut into diuerse parts, somewhat like unto the leaues of the knobbed Cranes bill, but larger, each of the cuts being larger and broader than they, which are cut in againe, so that the whole leafe being almost round, is halfe a foote long, and neere so broad also, set upon a foote stalke; an hand breadth long; from among which rise up, diuerse smooth greene crested stalkes, about two foote high, spread into branches, having finer cut leaues on them, and small pale yellow flowers at the toppes, with many threds in the middle, like unto others, after which cometh a small round knappe or head of seede.

The Place.
All these sorts of Crowfeete, doe grow in fields, meddowes, and arable grounds, many of them in our owne land, especially the first five sorts ; the rest by their titles may be understood from whence they came.

The Time.
The first and the great *Candye* sort are the earliest in flower, which is about March and Aprill, and the 13 and 14. are the latest that flower of all the rest, which is not untill September, all the other in May and Iune.

The Names.
It is called in Greeke βατράχιον, and there after in *Latine Ranunculus, non solum quia ranarum colorem folia multa imitantur, sed potius quia inter folia ranæ ut plurimum degunt :* in *English* we call them Crowfeete, rather than Frogwort after the *Latine,* from the divisions of the leaues, as I thinke, and therefore some call them *Pedes galli,* according to *Pliny,* yet some writers thought them to be *Coronopus pes corvi* of *Dioscorides,* and from thence
it

14. *Ranunculus autumnalis flore multiplici.*
Double flowred autumne Crowfoote.

Ranunculus Creticus latifolius.
Yellow broade leafed Crowfoote of *Candy.*

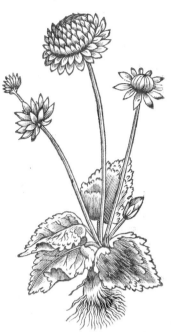
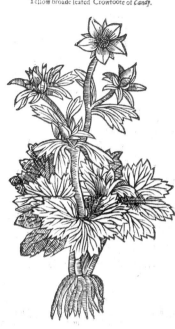

it is moſt likely our *Engliſh* name of Crowfeete came they have alſo diverſe other *Engliſh* namẽs, as King Cups, gold cuppes, Baſinets after the French, Piſſabeds, Bolts, Troll flower, and Locker Goulons, which two laſt are more proper to the eight kinde in my former Booke: of the *Italians Ranoncolo* and *Pie Corvino;* of the *Spaniards Yerva belida,* of the *French Grenoilette,* of the *Germanes Hanen fuſſ,* and of the *Dutch Hanen voet.* The firſt is *Tragus* his firſt *Ranunculus dulcis ſive pratenſis* by *Fuchſius Chryſanthemum ſimplex,* by *Dodonæus* in his *French* Herball and by *Lugdunenſis Polyanthemum ſimplex,* by *Tabermontanus Ranunculus dulcis,* & by *Bauhinus Ranunculus pratenſis erectus dulcis:* the ſecond is the *Ranunculus luteus* of *Tragus,* the *Ranunculus pratenſis ſurrectis cauliculis* of *Lobel,* & the ſecond *Ranunculus luteus* of *Dodonæus* & *Lugdunenſis.* *Thalius* calleth it *Ranunculus polyanthemus maculatus,* and *Gerard Ranunculus luteus* of *Dodonæus* & *Lugdunenſis.Thalius* calleth it *Ranunculus polyanthemus maculatus,* and *Gerard Ranunculus Batrachosides:* the third is called by *Lobel Ranunculus pratenſis reptante cauliculo,* by *Thalius Ranunculus polyanthemos primus,* by *Dodonæus* and *Lugdunenſis, Ranunculus hortenſis primus,* by *Tabermontanus Ranunculus vinealis,* and by *Bauhinus Ranunculus pratenſis repens hirſutus:* the fourth is called by *Lobel* in his *Icones Ranunculus arvorum,* as it is in the title, by *Dodonæus* and *Lobel* in his obſervations *Ranunculus ſylveſtris tertius,* by *Cordus* in his hiſtory of Plants, *Ranunculus ſegetalis,* by *Geſner in hortis Germaniæ Ranunculus arvenſis,* and by *Bauhinus Ranunculus arvenſis echinatus:* The fift is called by *Tragus Ranunculus exiguus & ſceleratiſſimus,* by *Geſner in hort Germaniæ Ranunculus Flammula, dictus,* by *Lobel Ranunculus bulboſus,* and by *Dodonæus tuberoſus,* by *Brunfelſius Crus Galli* and *Coronopus parvus;* it is generally taken to be, and ſo called *Batrachium Apuleij,* *Bauhinus* calleth it *Ranunculus pratenſis radice verticilli modo rotunda.* The ſixt is called by *Pona* in his *Italian* deſcription of Mount *Baldus, Ranunculus echinatus Creticus,* which he ſaith he had from *Signior Contarini* of *Venice,* *Bauhinus* calleth it *Ranunculus ſtellatus echinatus Creticus:* the ſeaventh is called by *Cluſius Ranunculus Apuleij quibuſdam,* *Pena* and *Lobel* ſet it forth in their *Adverſaria,* under the name of *Ranunculus paluſtris, rotundiore folio ſemine echinato,* but as *Bauhinus* ſaith in his *Phytopinax* and *Prodromus,* they confound it with the other *Ranunculus paluſtris rotundifolius levis* and therefore he calleth it *Ranunculus paluſtris echinatus,* not that it groweth in moorish ground but in wet fields. The eighth is called by *Bauhinus Ranunculus rotundifol. us repens echinatus.* The ninth is called by *Columna Ranunculus minimus Apulus,* as it is in the title, and by *Bauhinus Ranunculus arvenſis parvus folio trifido.* The tenth is called by *Cluſius Ranunculus Platophyllos,* and is his fift *Montanus,* which *Bauhinus* calleth *Latiſſimo folio hirſutus.* The eleventh is generally called of moſt writers, as alſo with all Herbariſts, *Ranunculus Illyricus minor,* and is the fourth *Ranunculus grumoſa radice* of *Cluſius,* and by *Bauhinus Ranunculus lanuginoſus anguſtifolius grumoſa radice minor.* The twelfth is called by all *Illyricus major,* being of the ſame kind, which *Bauhinus* therefore calleth, *Ranunculus lanuginoſus anguſtifolius grumoſa radice major,* and remembred by *Cluſius* in the ſame place with the other. The thirteenth is called by *Cluſius Ranunculus autumnalis,* and *Luſitanicus,* and is his firſt *Ranunculus grumoſa radice,* whereof he maketh two ſorts, and hath two figures upon the diverſities of the leaves and flowers, it is therefore called *Luſitanicus* by *Lobel, Dodonæus, Dalechampius* and all others, except *Bauhinus,* who calleth it *Ranunculus latifolius bullatus Aſphodeli radice.* The fourteenth is remembred by *Iacobus Cornutus* onely in his Booke of Canada plants. The fifteenth is called by *Bauhinus Ranunculus grumoſa radice folio Ranunculi bulboſi.* The laſt is called alſo by him *Ranunculus Geranij tuberoſi folio,* as it is in the title.   The

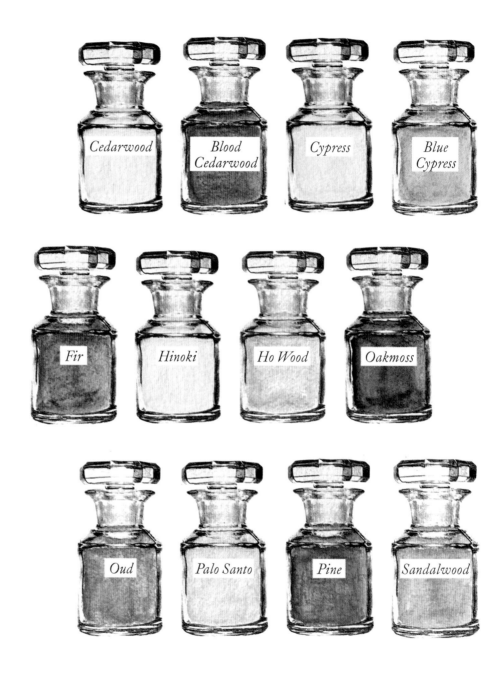

Cedarwood

Blood
Cedarwood

Cypress

Blue
Cypress

Fir

Hinoki

Ho Wood

Oakmoss

Oud

Palo Santo

Pine

Sandalwood

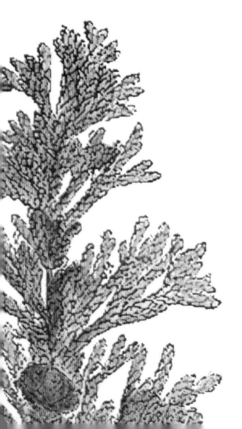

7
The Woods Family

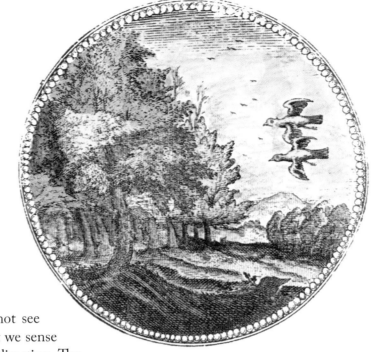

O nce we venture into the forest, we cannot see beyond the veil of trunks and leaves, but we sense the infinite journeys that lie down paths in any direction. The experience of the forest can't be fully captured in words or images, because it is made up of the richness of aromas, the mood of the light, the quality of the air, the interplay of solid trunks and spreading branches, the drama of upward motion, and our place inside that verticality.

Trees are the group of plants most akin to man, sharing not only our sense of uprightness but many body parts, like trunk, limbs, and crown. As we stand in the woods, we feel viscerally the diversity and immensity of nature. The essences of the forest remind us of these impressions. These fragrances concentrate our attention; smells bring you into a poetic moment: a rich experience that bridges from the present moment of smelling, sweeping you up imaginatively and pushing you toward a reverie.

With their roots in the ground, their limbs in the sky, and a lifespan that far exceeds our own, trees are a living symbol of the immortal. We feel this intuitively when we walk among them; standing under the canopy of ancient trees, inhaling their sweet, clean air, we are uplifted. When these aromas are distilled, the essences have a soft, warm note reminiscent of freshly cut wood.

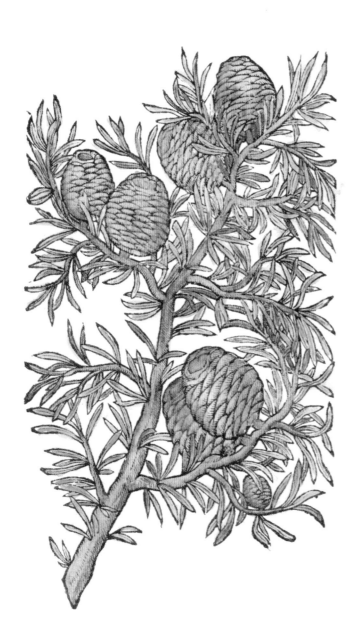

Cedar-wood

Juniperus virginiana

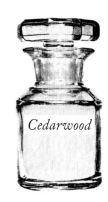

You will recognize this fresh, woody aroma immediately if you have ever chewed on a #2 pencil! The scent is memorably tied to cozy cabins and the winter storage of woolens in cedar chests: a homey, woody aroma that's soft, balsamic, and welcoming. Blood cedarwood, an essential oil derived from the heartwood, has a much more robust and intense smell—the deepest and warmest version, but still sweet. Cedarwood oil is seldom adulterated, because it is so inexpensive.

Available as various cedar essential oils.
Most useful are blood and Virginia.

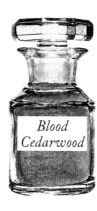

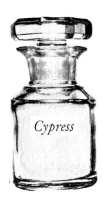

Cypress

Various *Cupressus* species

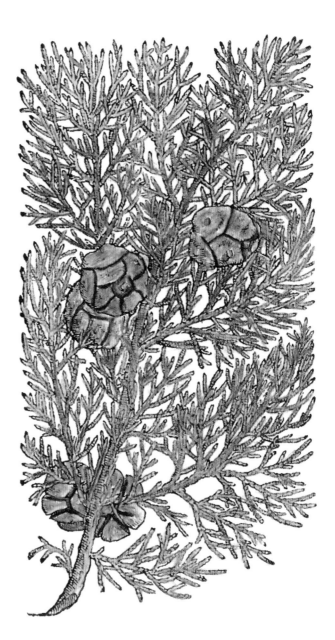

Known as "the mournful tree," Cypress was the symbol of grief in antiquity and was often planted in cemeteries. There is even an essential oil poetically named "weeping cypress." Cypress is associated with death because the tree fails to regenerate when it is cut back too much.

The airy, clean, dry aroma of cypress extends a feeling of openness and sea breezes. It is the unmistakable aroma of trees lining the ocean on the wild, craggy Big Sur coast of California.

Available as a clean, oceanic, and bright essential oil; as a dense, sweet absolute; and as a unique blue-colored essential oil from the blue cypress

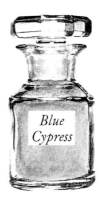

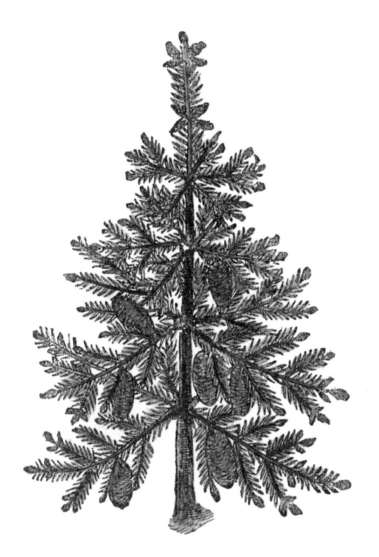

Fir

Various *Abies* species

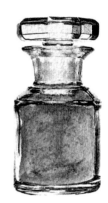

This refreshing coniferous aroma is bright, rich, sweet, and foresty. Reminding us of fresh Christmas trees, winter, and the holidays, the needles give off a delightful slightly citrusy scent. The whole tree is rich with aromatic balsam that accumulates on the bark and the tops of the cones. The smell is sweet and ambrosial—open, clean, rejuvenating.

Available as a sparkly essential oil
and a jammy rich absolute

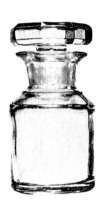

Hinoki

Chamaecyparis obtusa

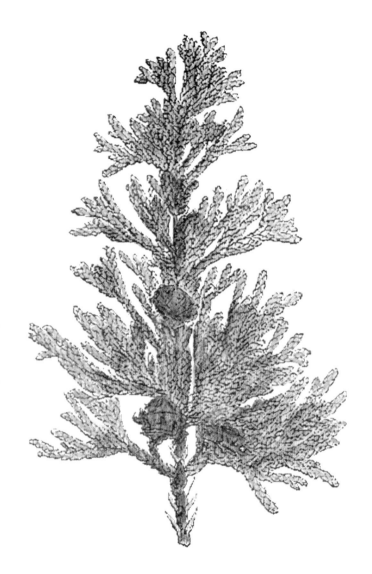

Hinoki is a species of cypress in Japan that grows where the air and water are pure. Hinoki wood has been valued since antiquity for the building of temples and Japanese soaking tubs. Groves of hinoki have been cultivated for *shinrin-yoku*, or "forest bathing," which is simply connecting with nature through our senses by being around trees. The essential oil is distilled from old stumps and roots, not from live trees. The light, woody, sweet, lemony aroma of hinoki is relaxing.

Available as an essential oil

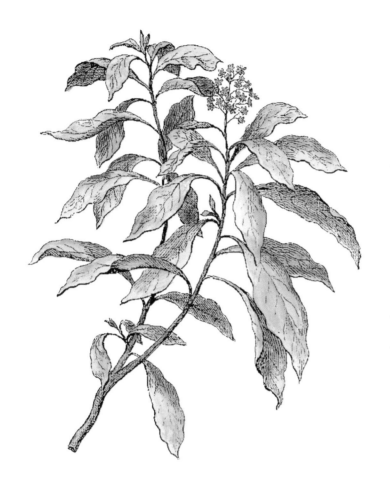

Ho Wood

Cinnamomum camphora

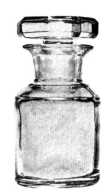

Steam distilled from the bark and wood of this evergreen tree, ho wood essential oil smells a lot like rosewood, but from a more sustainable source. An all-purpose top note, it blends easily with almost any other essence, adding a refreshing, light, rosy, sweet, woody aroma to the opening of a perfume. The essential oil has a vast amount of the dry floral aroma molecule linalool.

Available as an essential oil

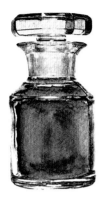

Oakmoss

Evernia prunastri

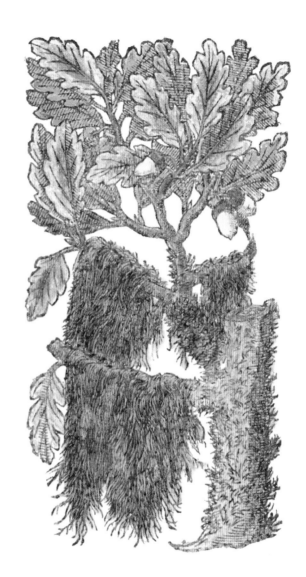

Oakmoss is a soft lichen, in undulating shades of green, that is collected from the branches and bark of oak trees. In its natural state, oakmoss has no discernible fragrance, but after it has dried and aged for a while, it develops a scent reminiscent of the seashore, bark, wood, and foliage. It is the rich and turgid smell of the wet forest, brush, and the underworld: dark, heavy, mysterious, loamy. The forest that fairy tales are set in—full of possibility, magic, and mystery. Incomparable and *sui generis*.

Available as an absolute

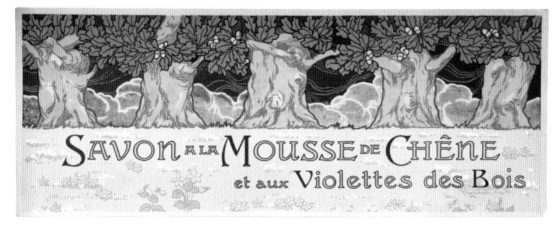

On this antique label for oakmoss soap, the trees look like they're straight out of The Lord of the Rings!

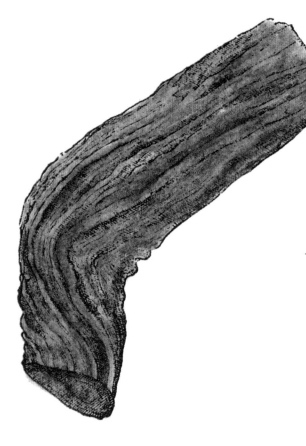

Oud

Aquilaria malaccensis
and related species

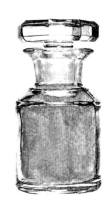

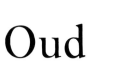

At $50,000 per kilo, oud is the most expensive of all essences. This highly fragrant wood comes from mature *Aquilaria* trees that are saturated with resin as the result of disease. Oud appears as veins or dark patches in the trunk and branches, distinct from the lighter, softer wood around it. Pieces of oud are graded by immersion in water: the best are the heaviest, which sink to the bottom, while poorer-quality pieces float. The Chinese called it "fragrance sinking underwater" or "sinking aromatic" and used it to drive out evil spirits and purify the soul. Oud's fragrance is complex, with an intense barnyard character. It is at once sweet and sour, spicy and animalic, earthy and woody.

Revered for incense through the ages, replicated synthetically but never very well, oud costs a scary fortune to purchase. Even when you have a lot of money to spend on it, it's very difficult to get a good specimen. Always imitated, never duplicated.

Available as an essential oil

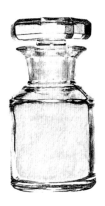

Palo Santo

Bursera graveolens

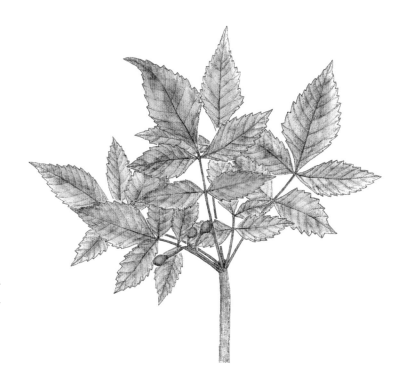

Palo santo means "holy wood," and this tree has long been used for sacred ceremonial purposes in South America. Palo santo oil is commonly distilled from the wood, but you can also find the rarer oil distilled from the fruit. The wood has more of a wintergreen facet, and the fruit smells fruity and woody.

Both wood and fruit are available as essential oils.

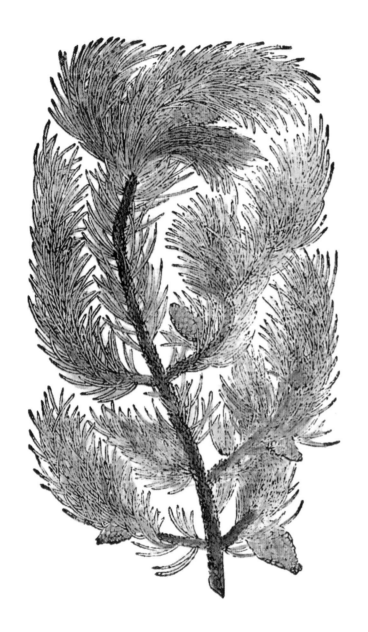

Pine

Various *Pinus* species

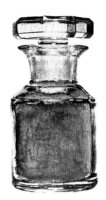

Pine trees reproduce with cones that contain male and female sex organs. The oldest known pine is 4,800 years old. The aroma of pine is, unfortunately, deeply associated with toilet-bowl cleaner. If you move away from that ubiquitous connection, you will find an aroma that is clean, piercing, and uplifting.

Available as various essential oils and an absolute. Scotch pine essential oil is bright and light, ocean pine essential oil smells like the sea air surrounded by trees, and pine needle absolute has a jammy, sweet, rich aroma.

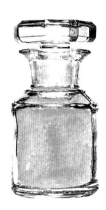

Sandal-wood

Santalum album

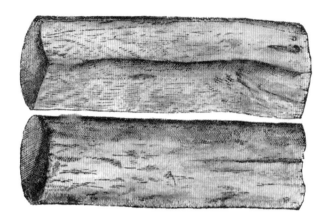

Sandalwood has been used as incense in various spiritual traditions for over four thousand years. In fact, its name derives from a Sanskrit word meaning "wood for burning incense." The essential oil develops in the tree after fifteen years and needs around another fifty years to reach full maturity. The best sandalwood oil comes from Mysore and Tamil Nadu in India and because of overharvesting is now protected by the state. Sandalwood's smooth, woody scent is calming and long lasting. The essential oil has no greeting note—the deep and low, sweet and milky aroma is unchanging and constant.

Available as an essential oil and as mitti, *a traditional version co-distilled with dirt. Mitti's aroma,* petrichor, *is the smell of dry earth plus fresh rain.*

Sandal, as found in the market, is the heart wood of the tree. After being felled, the bark is removed, the wood is cut in billets, and buried in the earth, in the native forest, for about two months, during which time the white ants eat off the outer layers, without touching the heart, which is the valuable portion. The pieces thus left are taken up and assorted according to their size and color. Their value increases with depth of tint; the deeper the yellow, the better the perfume. The old trees are, in all cases, most highly prized as the fragrance greatly increases with age.

—Snively, *Manufacture of Perfumes,* 1877

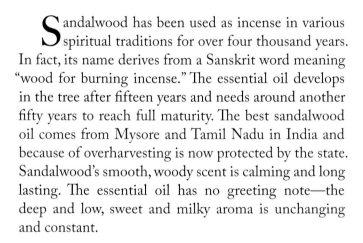

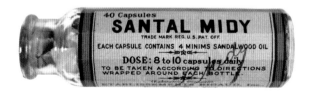

Hundred-year-old capsules filled with Mysore sandalwood. Take eight to ten daily!

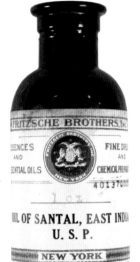

A full bottle of Fritzsche Brothers sandalwood from East India, early 1900s

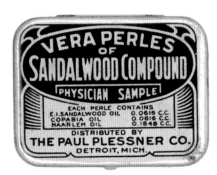

Sandalwood pills in a tin

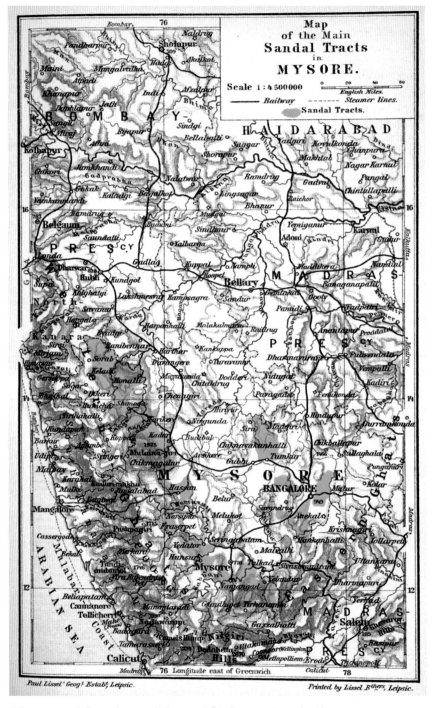

Mysore sandalwood map, Schimmel & Co. catalog, April 1900

8
Botanical Treasure Boxes

Imagination allows us to leave the ordinary course of things. Perceiving and imagining are as antithetical as presence and absence. To imagine is to absent oneself, to launch out toward a new life. . . . A true poet . . . wants the imagination to be a journey. *Every poet must give us his* invitation to journey. *Through this invitation, our inner being gets a gentle push, which throws us off balance, and sets in motion a healthy, really dynamic reverie. . . . This movement will not be a simple metaphor. We will really feel it within ourselves, most often as a release—as ease in imagining related images or desire to pursue a fascinating dream.*

—Bachelard, *Air and Dreams*

Botanical raw materials are the foundation of the Aftel Archive of Curious Scents! This is where everything begins and what everything is based upon. Perfection is inherent in the roots, barks, resins, woods, flowers, and seeds that yield the beauteous aromas. Just looking at the diverse and wondrous shapes, colors, and textures arouses our curiosity to know more about their use, lore, and history—and to find a way to include them in our lives. Some are from faraway places, and some are close to home; some thrive in the sunlight, and some live in the darkness underground. All are historically intertwined with us as people—across the globe and throughout time. Many are medicinal or sacred.

How better to share these treasures than in little drawers that beg you to open them with anticipation and desire? Little drawers have the quality of intimacy; the prospect of opening them carries the promise of discovery, secrecy, surprise: a treasure box. There is transgression, too, embodied in the act of opening drawers—rummaging through, fishing out, handling, caressing. Imagination carries the all-consuming desire to go deep into matter—touching and seeing and smelling! We long to dig in with our fingers, to reach the substance beneath superficial form and color—to touch the very heart of matter.

My museum features an antique tin-lined apothecary cabinet filled with materials that have been used for spiritual and medicinal practices since prehistoric times: balsams, resins, woods, leaves, roots, and flowers.

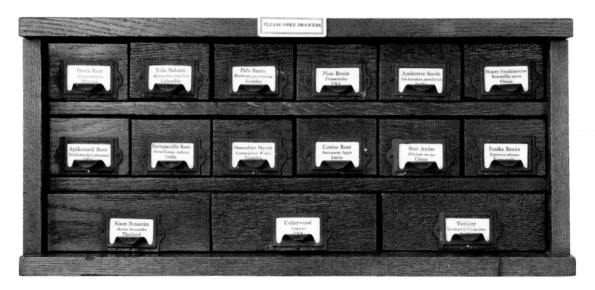

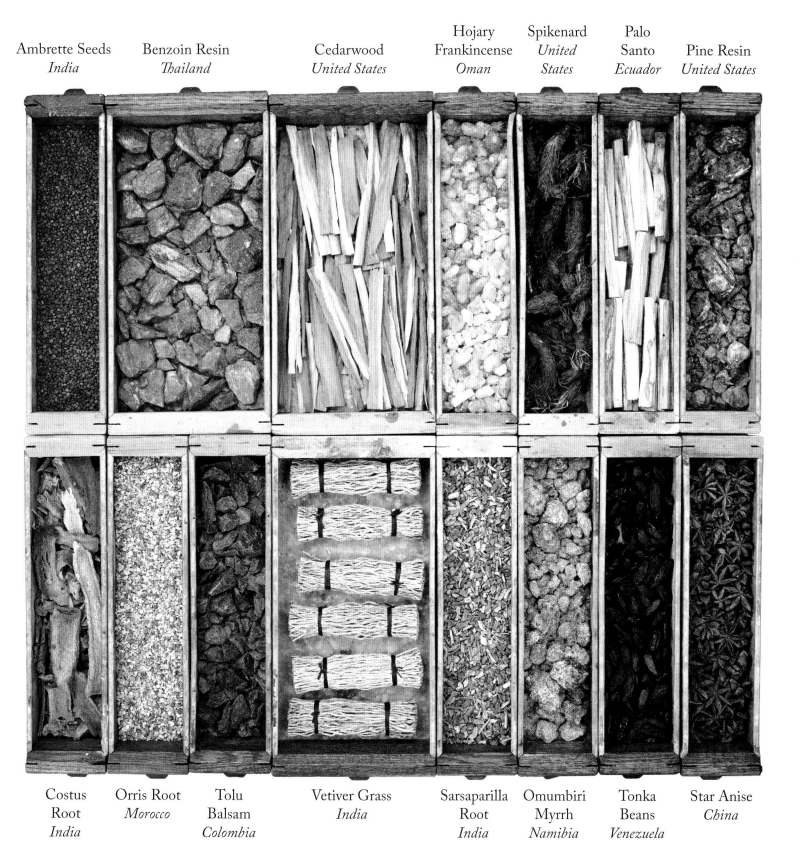

Ambrette Seeds
India

Benzoin Resin
Thailand

Cedarwood
United States

Hojary
Frankincense
Oman

Spikenard
United States

Palo
Santo
Ecuador

Pine Resin
United States

Costus
Root
India

Orris Root
Morocco

Tolu
Balsam
Colombia

Vetiver Grass
India

Sarsaparilla
Root
India

Omumbiri
Myrrh
Namibia

Tonka
Beans
Venezuela

Star Anise
China

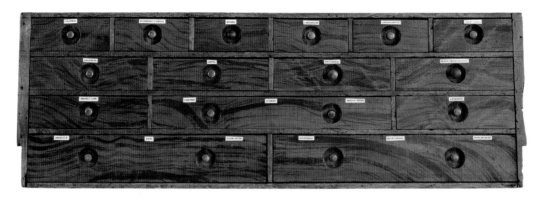

Watchmaker's oak cabinet from the 1830s, filled with raw materials for perfumery

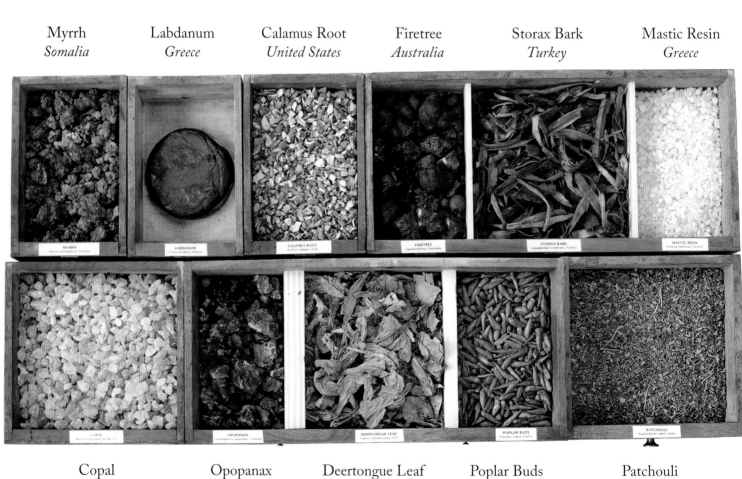

Myrrh
Somalia

Labdanum
Greece

Calamus Root
United States

Firetree
Australia

Storax Bark
Turkey

Mastic Resin
Greece

Copal
Mexico

Opopanax
Somalia

Deertongue Leaf
United States

Poplar Buds
France

Patchouli
India

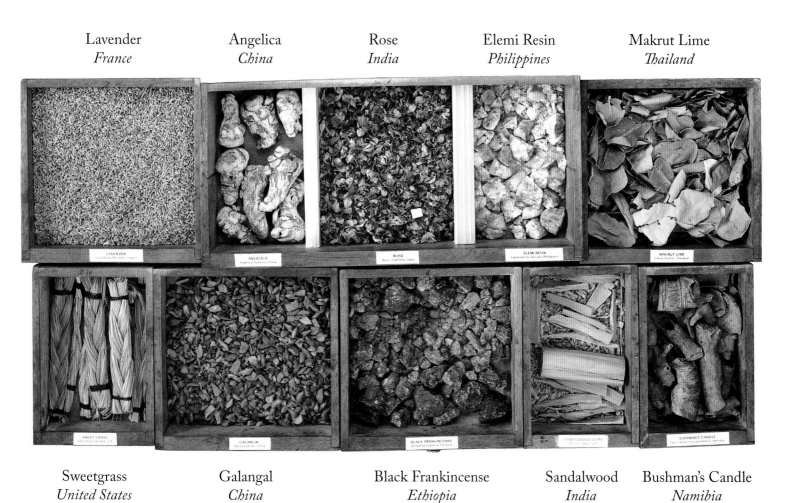

| Lavender *France* | Angelica *China* | Rose *India* | Elemi Resin *Philippines* | Makrut Lime *Thailand* |

| Sweetgrass *United States* | Galangal *China* | Black Frankincense *Ethiopia* | Sandalwood *India* | Bushman's Candle *Namibia* |

> Everyone should open up interior trap doors, journey into the depths of things, and let qualities invade. . . . Infinite indeed are the resources of the depths of things.
> —Francis Ponge, *The Voice of Things*, 1972

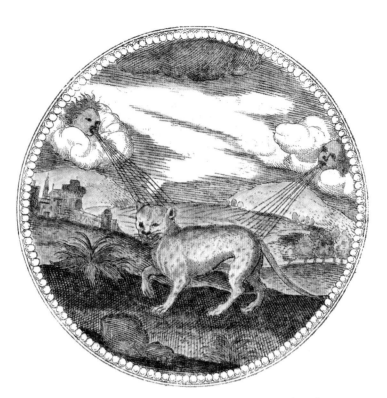

9
Civet

Give me an ounce of civet, good apothecary, to sweeten my imagination.
—Shakespeare, *King Lear*

The civet is a catlike animal with a long tail and a long, pointed muzzle like that of an otter. Its various species are native to Africa and much of Asia. The civet paste used for perfume is the potent secretion of the perineal glands of both males and females. Originally it was collected by killing the civet and removing the glands, but later the secretions of the live animal were harvested. Civet farming has involved animal cruelty in the past, but now people are trying to do it in a humane and sustainable way.

[Civet] is an excrementitious substance taken from a large double glandular receptacle, situated at some little distance beneath the tail of the civet cat. . . . Once a month, there is a sufficiency of this substance secreted for gathering; and then, by rubbing his tail against the wooden grate of his cage, the keeper knows that he wants to be civeted,—being in pain to get rid of the secreted substance. . . . This substance is of a yellowish colour, and of the consistence of an unguent.
—Lillie, *British Perfumer,* 1822

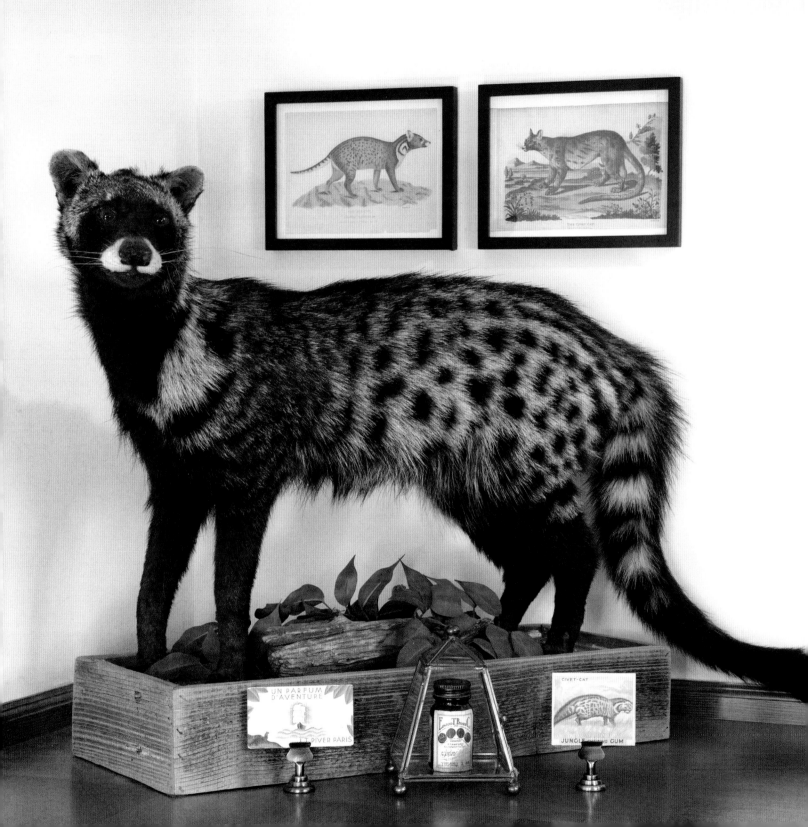

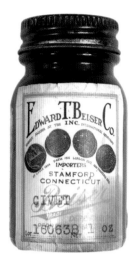

The aroma of civet embodies a yin-yang duality: in concentrated form, it is sultry and dirty—even fecal and nauseating—but when diluted it becomes beautifully floral, velvety, radiant, and narcotic. This duality is captured in the term "fecal-floral": the whiff of excrement this animal essence carries—as do some florals, like jasmine—gives it an unfathomable beauty, much more dimensional than pure sweetness could impart. Indole, a major component of civet, is responsible for this slippery slide from ugly to beautiful—from unpleasant to animalic to sweet—as it goes from highly concentrated to very diluted.

At a very high dilution [indole has] a pleasant flowery scent, recalling jonquil; when slightly stronger an element suggesting old clothes and sable fur comes in, which rapidly passes, with increasing concentration, into the smell of the lion house at the Zoo, and then into a frank stench. Even at its highest dilutions, when it is very sweet, this scent trembles on the edge of being unpleasant, for it lies very near the limit beyond which the nature of the stimulus becomes evident.

—Hampton, *The Scent of Flowers and Leaves*, 1925

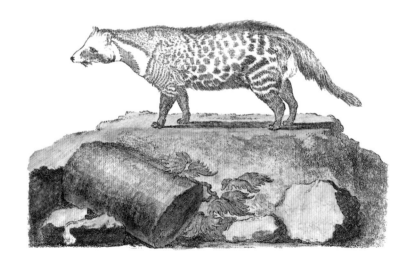

Civet is straight out of nature's cabinet of curiosities: it is a perfectly wondrous thing for this animal to contribute such a standout ingredient to perfume. It produces great effects in perfumes, smoothing out rough patches, adding a sense of shimmer, diffusion, and warmth. The aroma of civet is one of those weird and uncategorizable phenomena that stretch our understanding of what is possible. How on earth did people discover how to use this for perfume? Are there more things like it that we don't know about? It is like thinking about a distant planet and wondering if there are people on it.

Over the centuries, no five-star reviews
for the odor of civet

An extremely strong, and even unpleasant odour when fresh, so as sometimes to cause giddiness and head-ache.
    —Lillie, *British Perfumer*, 1822

In its pure state, civet has, to nearly all persons, a most disgusting odour.
    —Piesse, *Art of Perfumery*, 1857

Civet, in the natural state, has a most disgusting appearance, and its smell is equally repulsive to the uninitiated.
    —Rimmel, *The Book of Perfumes*, 1865

The odor is powerful, and in a concentrated state, extremely disgusting.
    —Snively, *Manufacture of Perfume*, 1879

Of all the animal substances used in perfumery, civet probably has the most revolting odor, closely resembling feces in this respect.
    —Perry, *Cyclopedia of Perfumery*, 1925

Just the odor is disgustingly obnoxious.
    —Poucher, *Perfumes and Cosmetics*, 1930

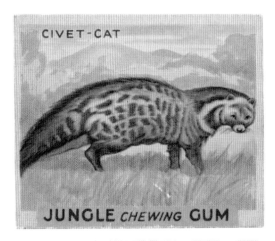

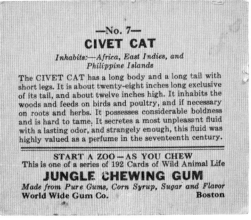

Civet chewing gum card

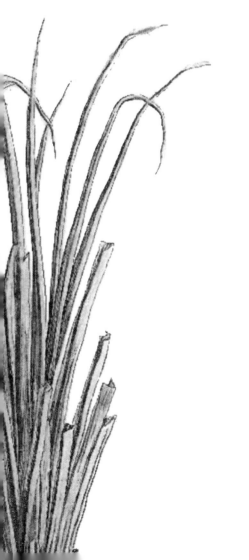

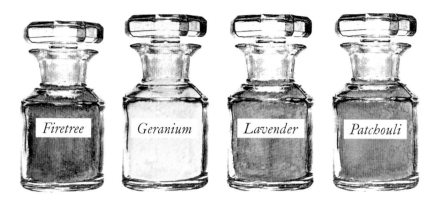

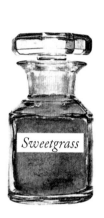
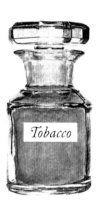
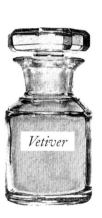
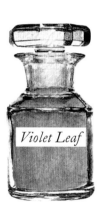

10
The Leaves & Grasses Family

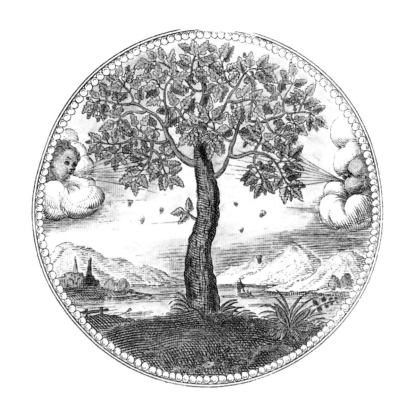

Essences from leaves and grasses are not like the more common aromas that come from culinary herbs. These essences are memorable, and woven into history and culture. They are polarizing as well—often people love or hate them. Leaf and grass aromas are rougher and more pungent than floral ones—sharp and refreshing, not delicate. They are also wildly different from each other, and they offer scent possibilities that are not to be found in any of the other fragrance families.

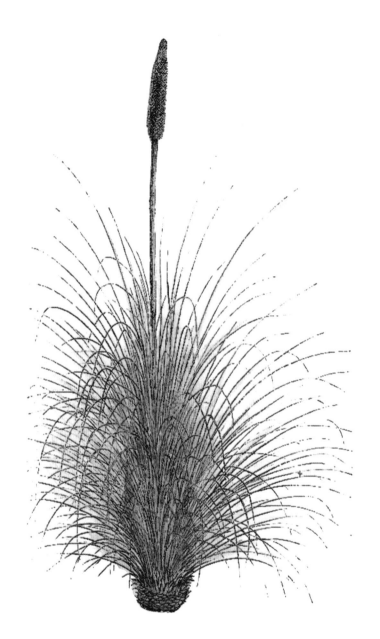

Firetree

Xanthorrhoea preissii

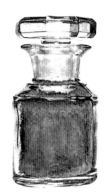

Firetree essential oil is distilled from the leaves of a most useful tree in Western Australia. Aborigines used the gum that oozes from the trunk to manufacture and repair weapons, the dry flower stalks to make fishing spears, the flowering spikes to flavor a sweet drink, and the tough leaves to cut meat.

One of the most tenacious essential oils, it shapeshifts aromas during its epic drydown. The aroma starts out as a very sweet floral (rose and lilac), then becomes a fruity balsamic, and finally a spicy, sweet, balsamic with notes of castoreum.

Available as an extremely rare essential oil

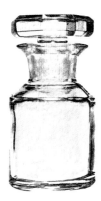

Geranium

Pelargonium graveolens

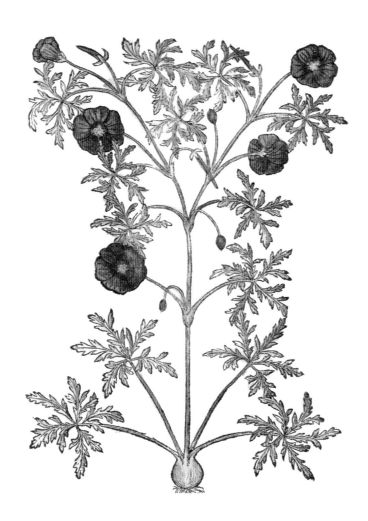

Geranium's essential oil is contained in small glands distributed over the surface of the leaves of the plant. These hairlike follicles are visible to the naked eye and give the surface of the leaves a silvery shine. When you press a leaf between your thumb and forefingers, you release the fresh, uplifting, rosy, leafy aroma.

This aroma is mostly geraniol and citronellol, which are also major components in rose. Geranium is often considered a "masculine" rose because it is fresher, greener, and less floral than actual rose.

Available as an essential oil

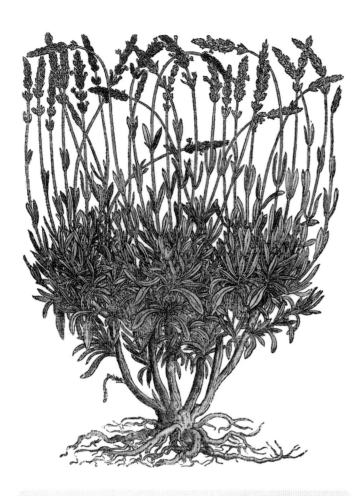

Lavender

Lavandula officinalis
(or *Lavandula angustifolia*)

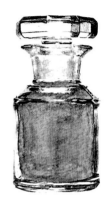

The word lavender is from the Latin *lavare*, which means "to wash." The best lavender is distilled from the plant when it is flowering (rather than budding or fading) and then aged for some time. Lavender aroma has balsamic-woody facets, a slight bitterness and spiciness—thanks to the presence of camphor. The most important components of lavender oil are linalool (floral) and linalyl acetate (fresh). Lavender absolute smells the most like flowers in bloom. As a bonus, the essential oil and absolute blended together in one perfume will enhance each other.

Available as an essential oil (thin, astringent, and sharp), as a concrete (smelling like soap), and in my favorite form—the gorgeous, turquoise-colored lavender absolute: sweet, spicy, and floral

The custom of preserving the petals of sweet-smelling flowers for the sake of their fragrant perfume is one of considerable antiquity.... We find in most old recipe books some method for preserving rose leaves and lavender, which were probably the earliest forms of pot pourri used in England. The very name of lavender is associated with cleanliness and freshness, and the old form of our "laundress" was "lavandre." The perfume of many of our sweetest flowers dies with them, and it is, therefore, obvious that only those which retain their odour when dried are of use in making a pot pourri. Of these the chief are the rose, lavender.

—C. J. S. Thompson,
The Housewife's Handy-Book, 1896

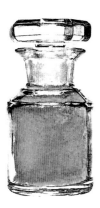

Patchouli

Pogostemom cablin

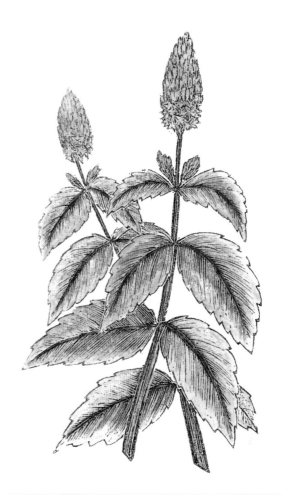

Patchouli is a dark brown oil distilled from the stems and leaves of the pogostemon plant, which resembles garden sage but with less fleshy leaves. For many, the smell of patchouli is wrapped in memories of the sixties. But back in the mid-nineteenth century, it was used to scent fine Indian paisley shawls to discourage moths from damaging them, and was also used for scenting India ink. A bag full of powdered dry leaves will both scent linen and repel moths.

The odor of patchouli is one of the longest-lasting of any botanical essence. Patchouli is the perfect balance of sweet, camphorous, woody, and musty (old coats) all at once. The aroma of patchouli imparts strength, character, and alluring notes to a perfume. The essential oil is most prized when it has been aged, as it grows richer over time. It has a sweet, rich, herbaceous top note and an earthy, slightly camphorous body note that evolves into a dry, woody, spicy note. Evocative descriptions of the aroma include old clothes, dry moss, and sable fur.

Available as an essential oil. The finest are aged.

Patchouli is a very shy flowerer, so much so that by the natives [of India] it is said to never flower; and Mr. Hardouin told me that though he had grown and bought it for the last thirty years, he had never seen or heard of such a thing as a flower.
—*Kew Bulletin*, June 1889

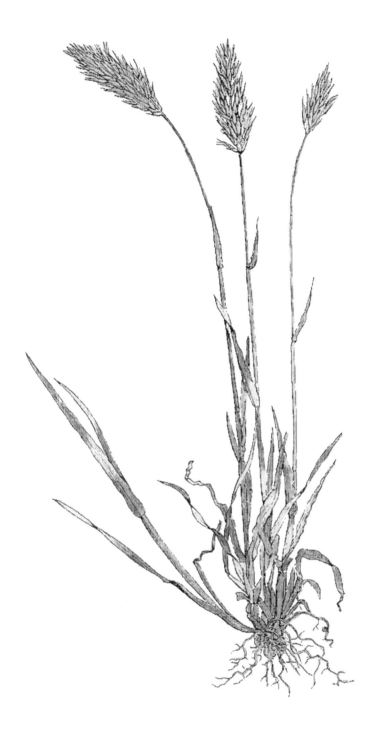

Sweetgrass

Anthoxanthum nitens
(or *Hierochloe odorata*)

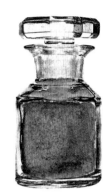

Many American Indian tribes use sweetgrass (also called vernal grass or flouve) in prayers and blessings. Considered a sacred plant, the grass is braided, dried, and burned as part of purifying ceremonies. The burning braid doesn't produce an open flame, but instead smolders and yields an attractive sweet scent that is used for smudging. The unlit braid may be offered at graves and sacred sites.

The powdery, tobacco-like aroma smells like fresh hay with a touch of vanilla. The sweetness comes from the aroma molecule coumarin.

Available as an absolute, called flouve: rich, complex, and of the countryside.

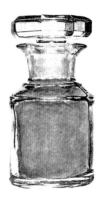

Tobacco

Nicotiana tabacum

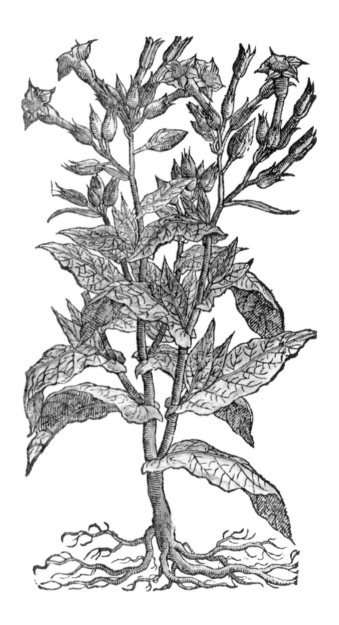

Tobacco, in the nightshade family, has been used by native peoples in healing and purification ceremonies. When tobacco leaves are cured, very few of them end up as raw materials for perfume.

When people think about the smell of tobacco, they usually have in mind a lit cigarette, where the aromas are transformed and dominated by the fire. The aroma of tobacco absolute, however, is musky, leathery, warm, and malty. Two important aroma molecules in tobacco leaf are guaiacol (smoky, whiskey) and phenylacetic acid (civet, floral).

Available as a nicotine-free absolute

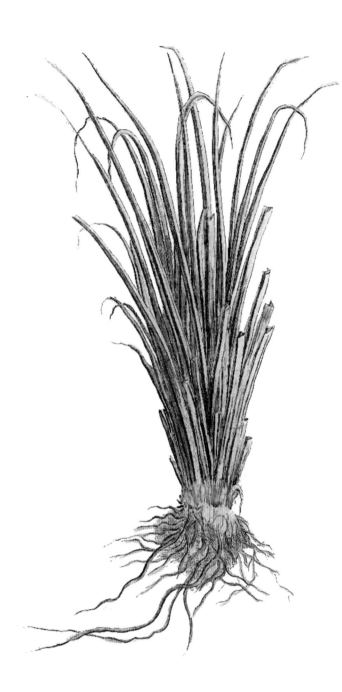

Vetiver

Chrysopogon zizanioides

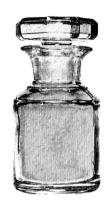

Vetiver's name comes from a Tamil word meaning "root that is dug up"; in northern India it is known as *khus*. The rootlets of this grass have been used for fragrance since ancient times. Dried vetiver has been used to scent linens and clothes. Woven into mats, sprinkled with water, and hung like curtains, vetiver creates a pleasant fragrance as it cools and scents the air in a dwelling.

The root possesses a soft, warm, rich aroma full of notes of grass, asparagus, precious wood, and wet soil. Older, thicker roots yield the best essential oil: fuller, richer, longer-lasting, and darker in color. Roots that have been stored for six months will require a long distillation process of thirty-six hours. Vetiver is aromatically a perfect complement to rose, adding the smell of stems and leaves to a rose fragrance.

Available as an essential oil

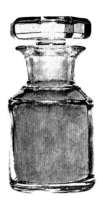

Violet Leaf

Viola odorata

Violet leaves are charmingly heart-shaped, and violet flowers have long been associated with tender emotions of the heart. The aroma of the flower—light, powdery, and "violety"—is much different than that of the leaves. Yet no violet scent would be complete without violet leaf absolute: distinctively green, earthy, and cool. This green leaf scent is powerful but also delicate; although not flowery, it brings up floral associations of bouquets of violets—including the leaves and stems—in the nose of the beholder.

Available as violet leaf absolute. The natural isolate alpha ionone smells like violets in bloom.

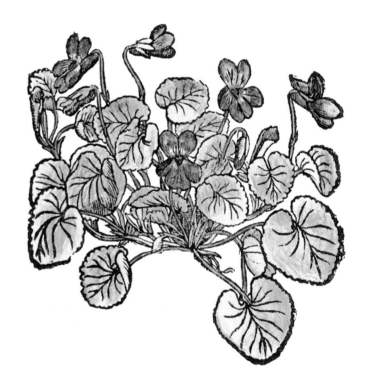

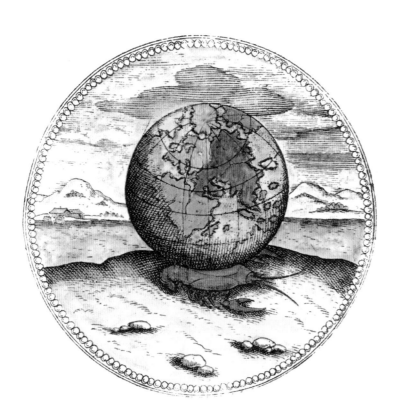

II
Beautiful Business

Natural essence suppliers at the turn of the century, like the Anton Chiris Company and Schimmel & Co., were not content with just extracting the most beautiful aromatics in the world. Inspired by these gorgeous essences, they seduced their customers with beautifully inventive hand-drawn maps, documentary photographs of people around the world gathering botanical materials, and fascinating information about the lore and chemistry of the essences themselves.

The Antoine Chiris company, founded in Provence in 1768, was a very successful supplier of quality natural raw materials for perfume. In the early twentieth century, they supplied François Coty's groundbreaking perfume company in Paris. Besotted with essences, Chiris created these fanciful maps that depict the world being discovered in perfume's wake. The maps include musk deer (musk), whales (ambergris), trees being tapped for resin, several sea monsters, and ships that sail across the dangerous waters to faraway places. The Africa map includes a compass dial listing the essences from there: vetiver, clove, ylang ylang, geranium, lemongrass, vanilla, citronella, and cinnamon. (The exploitation and racism inherent in many essential oil businesses were *not* beautiful!)

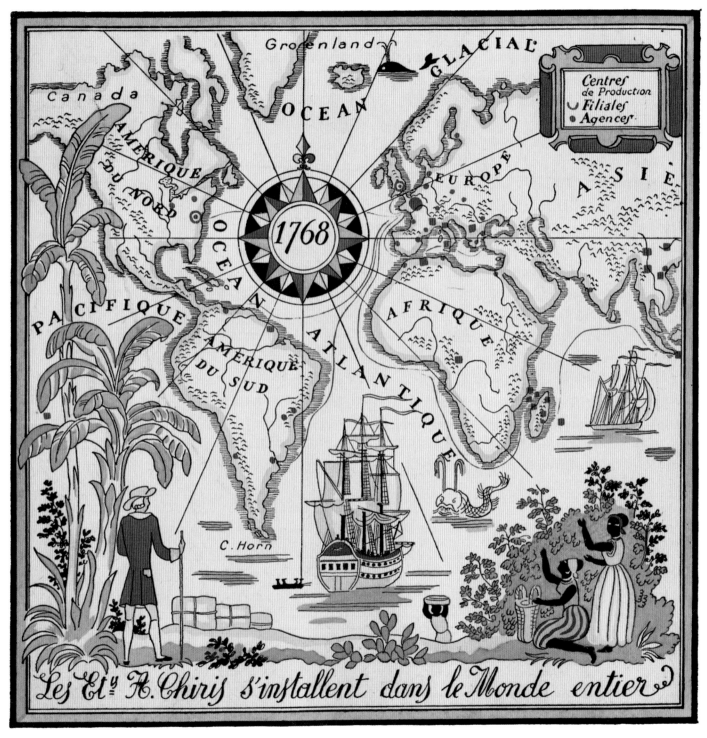

Chiris perfume map, 1931. This map and the ones on the following pages illustrate not only the global nature of the trade in natural essences but also its ties to colonialism.

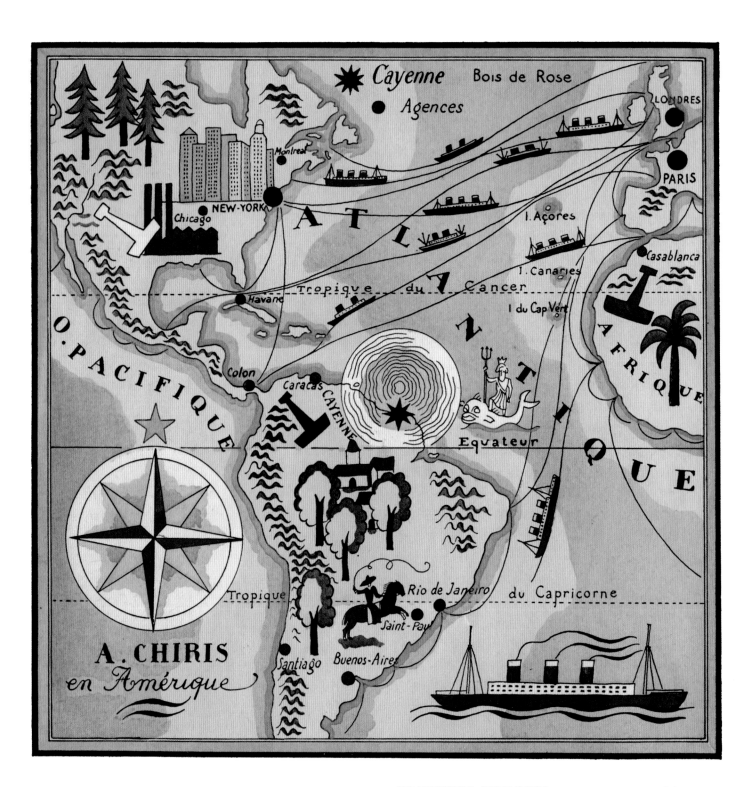

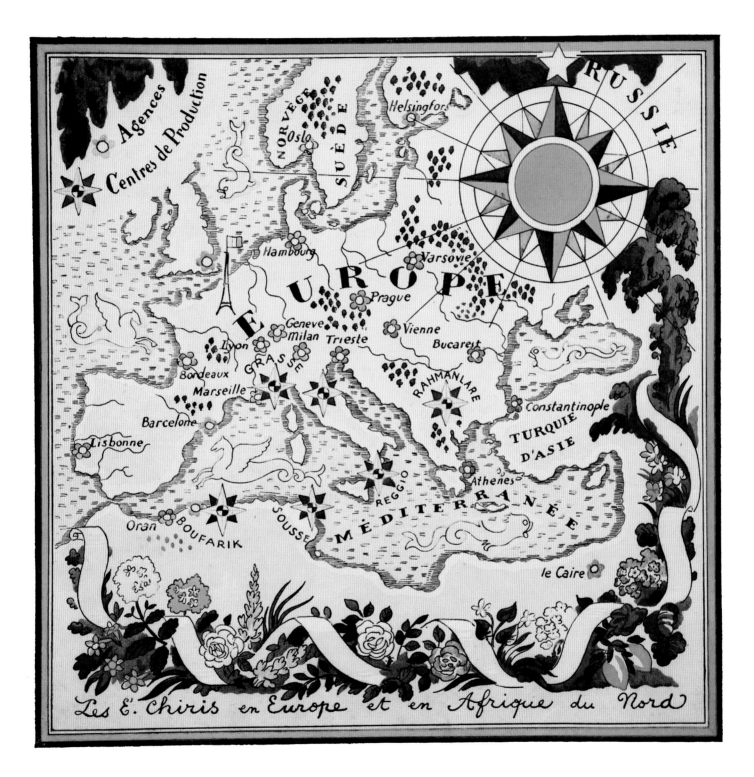

Les E. Chiris en Europe et en Afrique du Nord

BEAUTIFUL BUSINESS

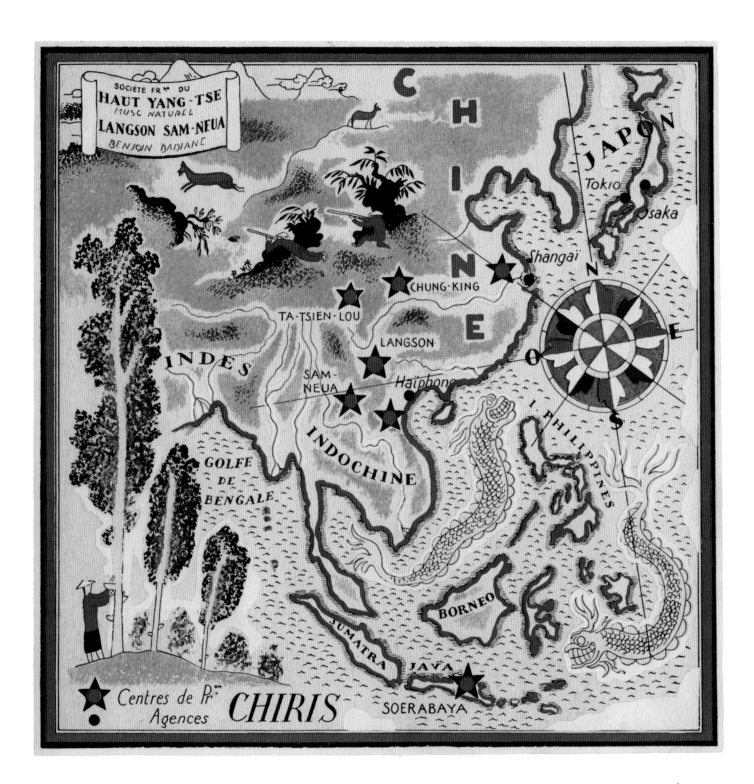

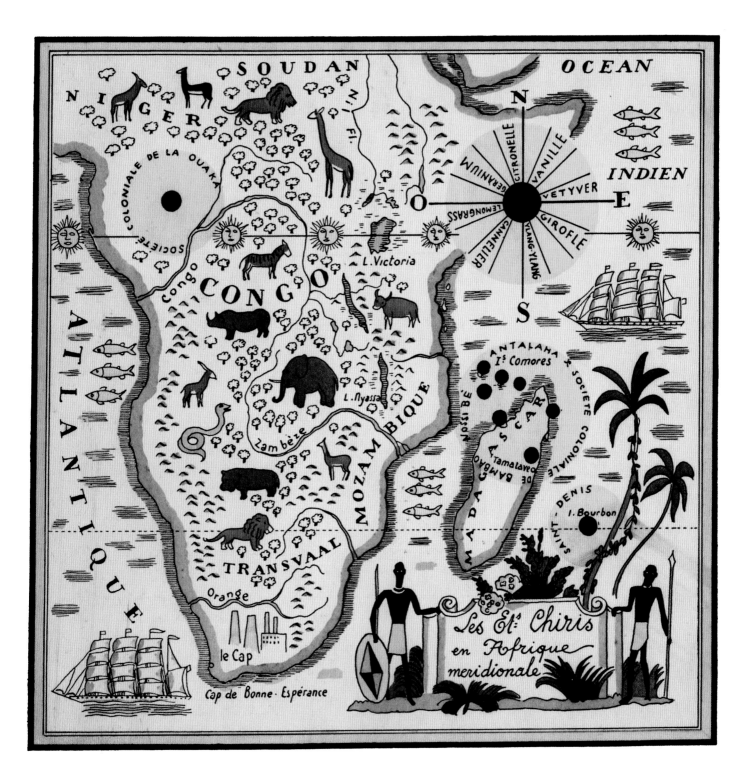

BEAUTIFUL BUSINESS

Schimmel & Co. of Leipzig, along with its American subsidiary Fritzsche Brothers, was the largest essential oil purveyor in the world, and their twice-yearly catalogs were a treasure trove of maps, illustrations, and photographs of aromatic materials and essential oils from many lands. These incredible catalogs, running from 1887 to 1915, chronicle the discovery of natural essences across the globe. The writing is vibrant with accounts of history and exploration, sometimes in countries that have since disappeared or been absorbed. The catalogs include many hand-colored maps, photos of people harvesting botanicals, precise details of sandalwood auctions, and flights of fancy off the beaten track. They also helped establish essential oil chemistry as a scientific field, detailing methods and standards.

Here are a few selections from the catalogs.

Peppermint—Menthol   *October 1901*

The exceptionally hot summer in Europe and America has exerted a powerful influence on the consumption of this prominent refreshing medium and has also brought the useful migraine pencils back into favour. Menthol is nowadays used for such a variety of purposes, that it has long since lost the character of an article of fashion and has entered the ranks of indispensable medicaments. The preparations and specialties for which it is employed are legion.

Camphor Rituals   *April 1905*

H. Furness, who has lived for a long time in Borneo and has studied the habits of the "head-hunters," describes these in an attractive manner, and we do not consider it out of place to give some details on the ceremonials which must be observed in gathering the camphor.

When the "Kayans" are about to undertake a search for the trees which are to supply them the valued camphor, they first of all make very careful observations of certain external occurrences which they consider as good or evil omens for the result of their undertaking. It is especially the flight of certain birds, such as the spider-hunter, the red hawk, or the rainbird, on which the result of the search depends. If they see one of these birds cross their path from right to left, there is

SEMI-ANNUAL REPORT
of
SCHIMMEL & Co.
(FRITZSCHE BROTHERS)

LEIPZIG. NEW YORK.
LONDON.

OCTOBER 1900.

SEMI-ANNUAL REPORT
on
Essential Oils,
Synthetic Perfumes, &c.
Published by
SCHIMMEL & Co
(Fritzsche Brothers)
MILTITZ
near Leipzig
LONDON —— NEW YORK

OCTOBER 1914 / APRIL 1915.

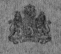

Sandalwood auctions 1911.

The districts of production of
Lavender- and Spike oil
in
SOUTHERN FRANCE.
Scale 1:1500000

Legend:
Lavender oil, ordinary, fine.
Spike oil.

GOLFE DU LION   MARSEILLE

Map of the
Clove Districts
of
ZANZIBAR AND PEMBA.
Scale 1:800000

English Miles

Clove districts

ZANZIBAR

ISLAND

GERMAN   ZANZIBAR CHANNEL

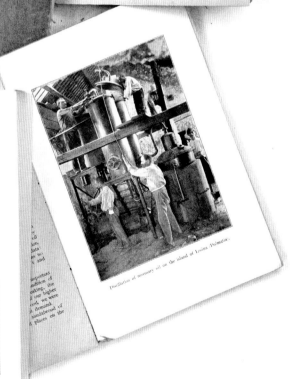

Distillation of rosemary oil on the island of Lesina (Dalmatia).

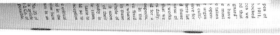

In our last Report we published an illustrated description of the
distillation of palmarosa oil in the district of Amraoti, British India
Mr. I. H. Burkill, of Calcutta, to whom we were indebted for the in-

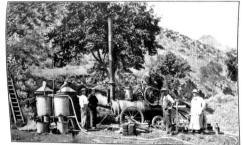

Schimmel & Co.'s itinerant Lavender distillery at Castellane.

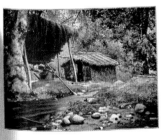

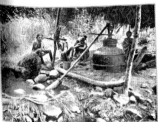

Distillation of Palmarosa oil at Kandesh (British India).

but small prospect of a good haul; but if they see the birds fly in the opposite direction, they consider it a portent of a good result of their expedition, and only when the omens are satisfactory do they proceed on their way. But before the work can be commenced, they must hear the trot of a stag, and finally must kill a certain kind of snake. Only when all this has taken place, they may hope to find a rich harvest.

When all the signs are favourable for the camphor hunters, and if the tree is found to contain a sufficient quantity of camphor, a post is erected which is clothed with chips and brushwood (the chips are possibly intended to represent the sinuous tongues of fire which are connected with the invisible powers). During the gathering of the camphor the "Kayans" are allowed to take food, and to speak to people whom they meet, but no stranger is allowed to enter their hut. When the tree is felled, it is cut up in small pieces by the hunters, who for this purpose dress themselves in fine clothes and put on arms. They therefore consider it as a fallen enemy, of whose hidden treasures they can only possess themselves by means of sword and spear. The search for crystals is extremely troublesome, as every piece of wood has to be cut up small and tested with the greatest care.

The Odor of Sanctity *April 1908*

The "odour of sanctity" was not a merely metaphorical expression with old writers. In Malory's "History of Prince Arthur," written in the fifteenth century, we find that when the wicked Sir Corsabrin's head was cut off, "therewithall came a stench out of the body when the soul departed, so that there might nobody abide the savour." This was at the time supposed to be the disodour of the unbaptized. But when his comrades found Sir Launcelot dead, they noticed "the sweetest savour about him that ever they smelled," which Malory describes as the odour of sanctity.

Usually the saintly odour is compared with the odour of violets, cloves, orange blossoms, lilies, roses, cinnamon, pineapple, yellow amber, and benzoin.

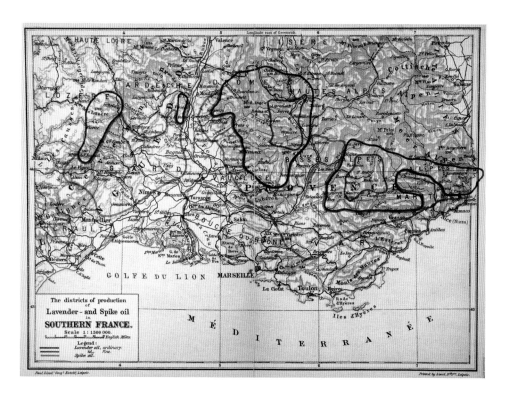

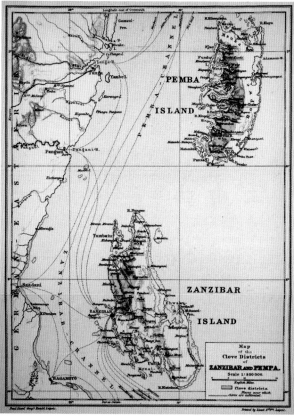

ABOVE

Map of lavender production in southern France, Schimmel & Co., April 1899

LEFT

Map of clove production on Zanzibar, Schimmel & Co., October 1900

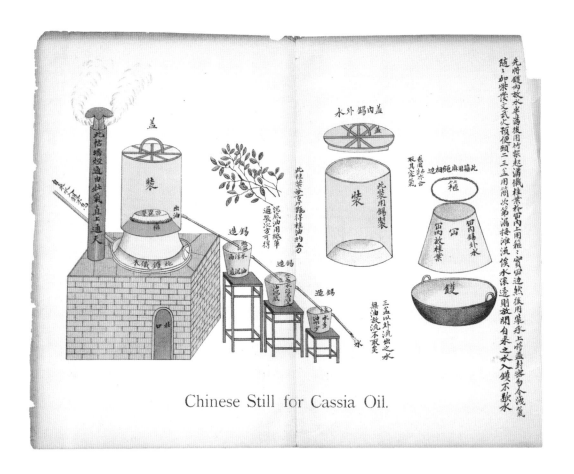

先府鐵內放水半滿後用竹架起溝放桂葉於內用糍以實當邊然後用裝承上將蓋封落勿令漏氣
隨、加柴猛又武火預使頸二三盞用間次第漏遑流後水漾透則放開自垂之水入鑊不歇水
水外鍚內蓋

此桂葉要宗跪得桂油約分

此樓用鍚製

裝

蓋

裝

造鍚

造鍚

造鍚

此怙蠄煙過由牡氣直上通天

沉底油用鉛筆過氣沉方可得

衣儀鐘此

邊相絕麻用織此取其落氣

箱

瓦內鍚外水

瓦內放桂葉

鑊

三盞以外流出之水無油放流不限矣

水

Chinese Still for Cassia Oil.

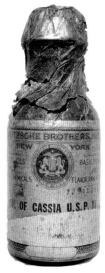

Tzsche Brothers
New York
Basic
Chemicals Flavor Raw
Oil of Cassia U.S.P. XI

This beautiful drawing of a cassia still with Chinese calligraphy—and even smoke coming out of the smokestack—appeared in the 1895 Schimmel catalog. Cassia oil comes from a relative of cinnamon with a similar aroma, but more like Red Hots candy than the sweet woodiness of cinnamon itself.

This bottle of oil of cassia in my museum is from the same timeframe as the Chinese still drawing, filled with exactly the material that was being extracted. The bottle feels magical, with its old paper cover that has never been unwrapped and a beaten metal top sealed over the cork. It is filled with a pungent essence that was last smelled over a hundred years ago, bottled up like a genie.

These picturesque postcards of itinerant distilling at the turn of the century show large mounds of botanical material. You can almost smell the air redolent of fresh fragrance—a beautiful process and beautiful images in harmony with nature.

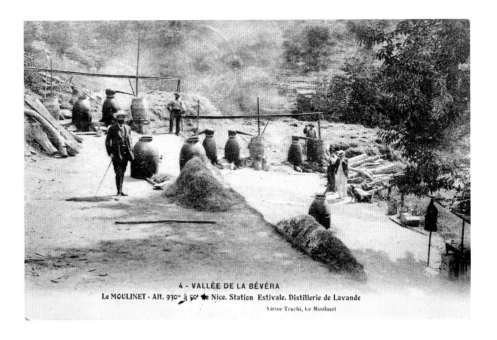

4 - VALLÉE DE LA BÉVÉRA
Le MOULINET - Alt. 930ᵐ à 50ᵏ de Nice. Station Estivale. Distillerie de Lavande
Victor Truchi, Le Moulinet

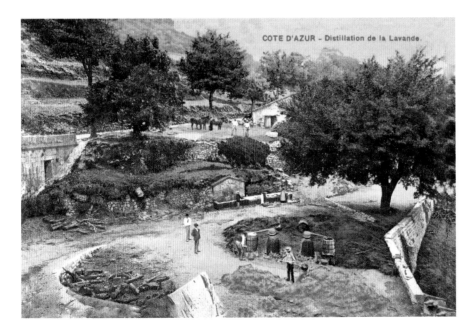

COTE D'AZUR - Distillation de la Lavande.

Both scenes show the distillation of lavender—one of the botanicals most commonly distilled in the south of France. An example of the locavore connection to plants and the importance of terroir.

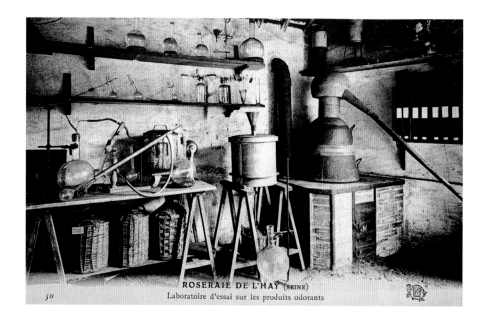

ROSERAIE DE L'HAY (SEINE)
Laboratoire d'essai sur les produits odorants
50

The passion for aromatic plant essences was so widespread that some people had still rooms in their own homes where they distilled fragrant plants.

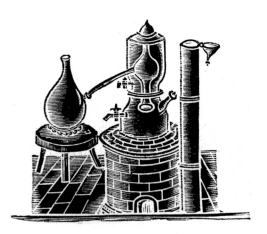

Woodcut from The Still Room

The still-room was a most important apartment in every country-house of any size. No housewife's education was complete without a knowledge of the still and the process of distillation, by means of which she prepared her aromatic waters, dried her herbs and simples, prepared her wines, cordials, syrups, and the many other excellent products which the still-room furnished. . . .

We can picture the still-room as it was a hundred or more years ago. A long, low, rambling sort of place, with many odd nooks and corners, and lit by narrow windows. Beneath the benches are wine kegs, stone jars, and mash tubs, and the shelves, which run from end to end of the opposite wall, are lined with bottles, jars, and pots, all neatly labelled.

In the further corner stands the still, beneath whose bulb a low red fire glows, and from its neck the fluid drops like liquid amber into the glass receiver. Small alembics, with tall glass jars, repose beside it. Close by is the marble mortar on a stout four-legged stand, for pounding knotty roots and other hard bodies.
—C. J. S. Thompson, *The Housewife's Handy-Book*, 1896

Filled with possibilities, this was the glorious history of a thriving industry that made natural ingredients for perfume. The beauty inherent in the process of creating the oils parallels the beauty inherent in the plants themselves. Beauty begets beauty. The resulting essential oil was born from a deep care for the minute ministrations that yielded the aromatic potential of flowers, leaves, and grasses. We can feel the passion of the people working with these materials as they bottled up their essences, a passion that in turn inspired perfumers to include them in their creative practice. The magic and beauty in these bottles were the foundation of everything created in the world of perfume. However, this reliance on gorgeous natural essences came to a close in the middle of the twentieth century.

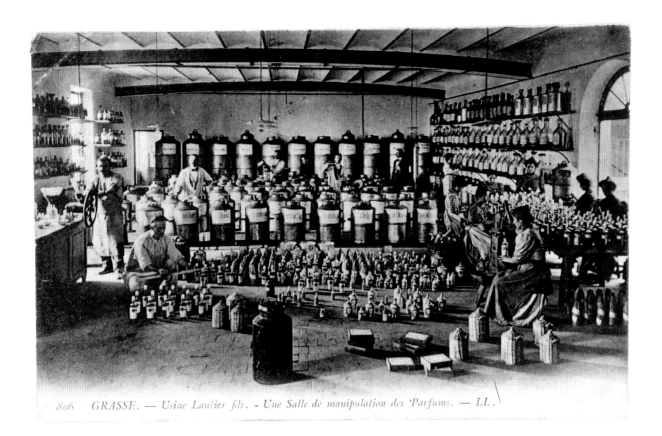

806   GRASSE. — Usine Laulier fils. - Une Salle de manipulation des Parfums. — LL.

Here in the Aftel Archive of Curious Scents, these mysterious, turn-of-the-century bottles are filled with their original aromatic essences. They contain the whole world of exploration inside their glass walls. The bottles present a collage of blue and amber glass, with their sloping shoulders covered in dust and labels ranging from ragged to pristine, printed in a medley of fonts. Sometimes there are metal beading and stamped seals around the cork, or the bottle itself is covered in paper.

Inside each bottle, captured over a century ago, the essential nature of the plant is still energetically alive. Even without opening the bottle, we are aware that we are in the presence of a powerful kind of purity, beauty, strength—the life force of the plant has stayed bottled up, like a hundred-year-old genie in a lamp. These essences were once alive and radiate that vivacity. Like a spirit or a being imprisoned in matter, the shapeless aromas themselves serve as a sort of psychic, subjective

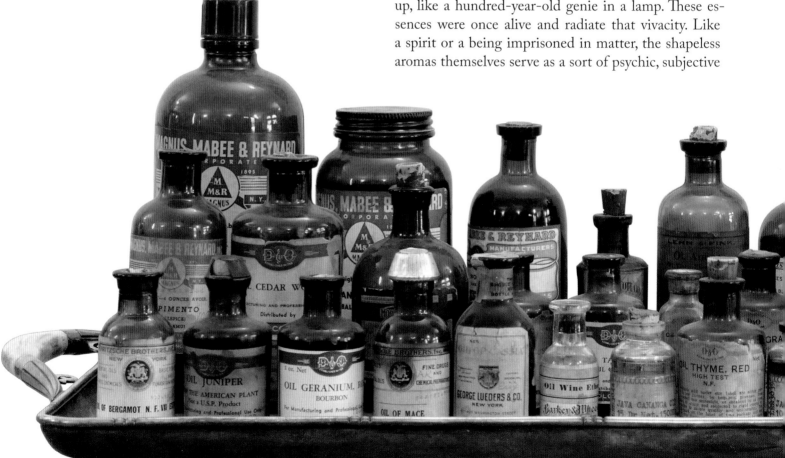

complement to the external forms of atoms, cells, and plants. Because the bottles have not been opened, they are more mysterious than if they were. They are inviolate. They have a magic, a promise of suspended discovery that hasn't happened (yet).

When you peer into the glass, you see the oils, some having thickened over time, like syrup. These bottles are decontextualized—their context was to be in labs, pharmacies, perfume businesses. You look at them and wonder, where have they been? What have they been used (or not used) for? Fantasizing about their previous lives creates a sense of wonder.

Objects have itineraries: we meet them at one point in their travels, informed by where they have been. The very names of the essences are transporting. People use them in poetry, songs, and literature to evoke moods: the earthy, the fine, the sensual, the exotic, the timeless. They have an internal life and magic, an ability to transport from where they have been.

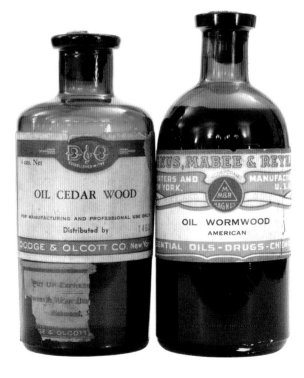

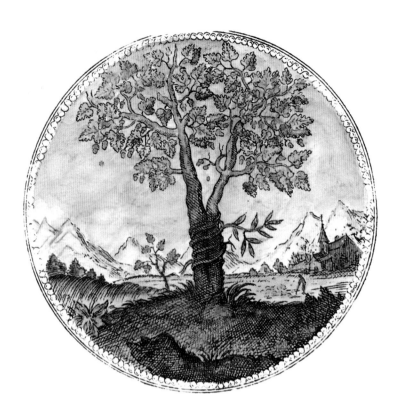

12
Wood of the Gods

The resin-permeated heartwood of *Aquilaria* trees, known as *oud* or *agarwood*, is the most expensive wood in the world, because of its complex and beautiful aroma. An immune reaction to a fungal infection causes the tree to produce a fragrant oleoresin, which is deposited in irregular dark streaks inside the wood. The fungi usually occur in trees over fifty years old. There are more than 150 fragrant molecules that constitute agarwood's highly complex aroma. The specific character of the aroma depends on a combination of factors: the region where the tree grows, its species, its age, the part of the tree from which the wood is taken, and the amount of time the wood has undergone the biochemical process.

The enigmatic origins of agarwood have given rise to myth and legend. The ancient Egyptians are believed to have been the first users of oud, in funerary rituals more than three thousand years ago, and it was a valuable commodity on the ancient trade routes. Agarwood is mentioned twice in the Old Testament, in Numbers and Psalms.

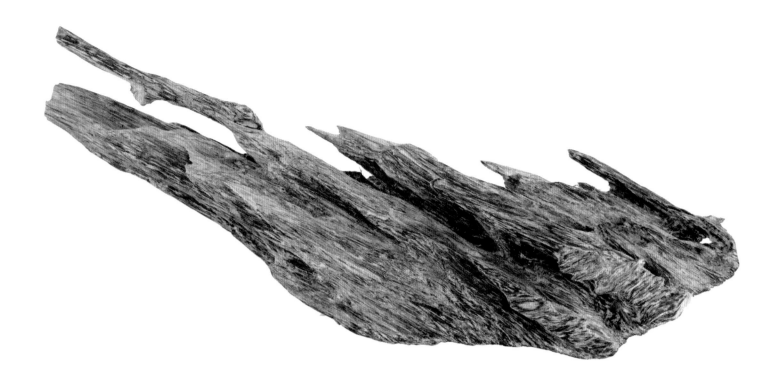

Agarwood is sold in various grades depending on the resin content, specific gravity, odor, and color. The frequency of natural infection is low and a matter of chance, and even on *Aquilaria* plantations only 7 to 10 percent of the trees ultimately form resinous oud. The phenomenon of natural agarwood formation has yet to be completely understood.

Over the past fifty years, there has been a dramatic increase in the demand for oud. Due to the rampant destruction of natural habitats, most oud-bearing trees are considered endangered. Since most of the agarwood trees grow in wild areas, there is great concern for their sustainability. The global trade in agarwood is around 7 billion dollars a year, making it the most commercially valuable plant species in the world.

A five-ounce piece of Sabah oud from northern Borneo, Malaysia, donated by KyaraZen. It has a rich aroma, with notes of fruit, spice, incense, and the jungle.

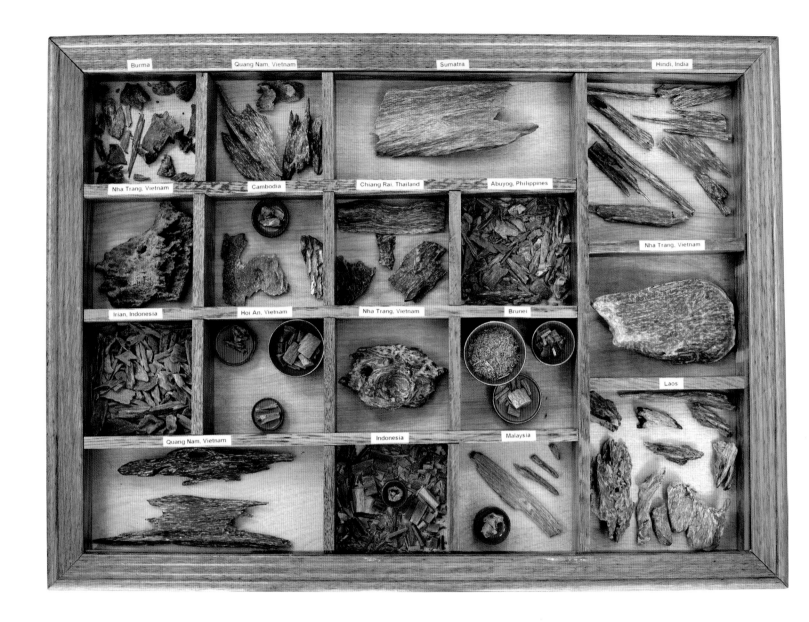

Burma

Quang Nam, Vietnam

Sumatra

Hindi, India

Nha Trang, Vietnam

Cambodia

Chiang Rai, Thailand

Abuyog, Philippines

Nha Trang, Vietnam

Irian, Indonesia

Hoi An, Vietnam

Nha Trang, Vietnam

Brunei

Laos

Quang Nam, Vietnam

Indonesia

Malaysia

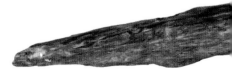

The collection of small oud pieces pictured opposite was left to the Aftel Archive by the master incense maker Ross Urrere and is displayed in his memory. It includes specimens from Brunei, Cambodia, India, Indonesia, Laos, Malaysia, Myanmar, the Philippines, Thailand, and Vietnam.

Below is a ten-ounce pice of Sasoura oud from India, generously donated by KyaraZen and friends of Ross Urrere. Sasora is one of the six categories of oud designated in sixteenth-century Japan, based on geographical origin as well as sensory-spiritual knowledge. This forty-year-old piece, harvested from a tree that was over a century old, is "half sinking" with good resination. The aroma is initially cooling, followed by a deep sweetness that is not cloying but stoic and, in some way, reminiscent of a Zen monk.

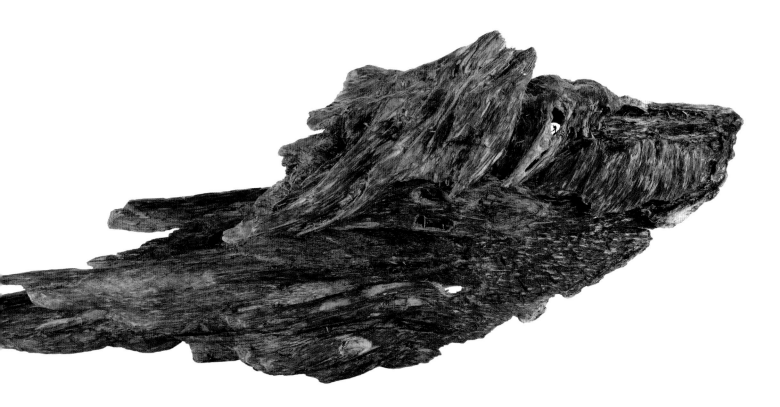

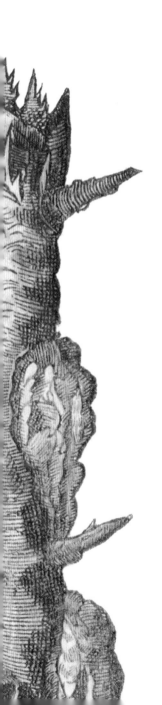

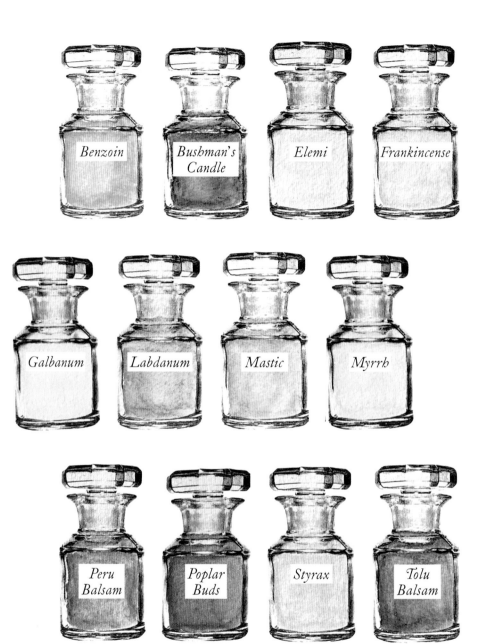

13 The Resins Family

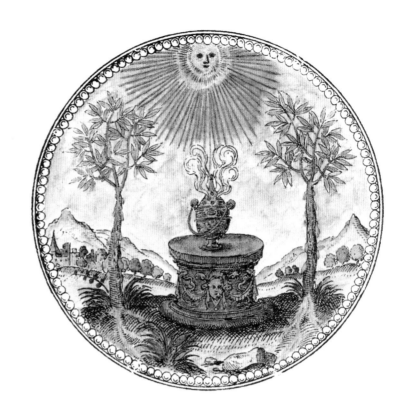

Spirit is the heart of matter;
matter is the ensoulment of spirit.
   —Bachelard

R esins are fragrant exudations from trees and plants, typically a thick aromatic sap that hardens into crystals. They look like jewels, and when you handle them, they transfer their perfume to your skin. They are of great use to the perfumer for their staying power.

The word *perfume* comes from the Latin *per fumum*, "through smoke," and the original perfumes were incense. Resins—flammable and good-smelling as they are—have long been used as incense and incorporated into the rituals and belief systems of many religions. With their complex aromatic layering, these substances are a vehicle for spiritual exaltation. Burning incense opens a door between the mundane and the supernatural; its aromas contain compressed time for the person smelling them. Resins, passionately adopted and patiently explored, provide an opening in every sense of the word.

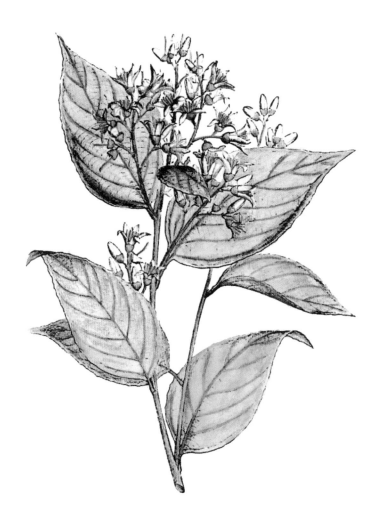

Benzoin

Styrax benzoin

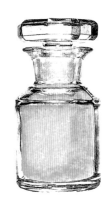

Benzoin resin is a pathological secretion—when the trees are allowed to live normally, they don't produce benzoin. The infliction of a sufficiently deep wound to the tree results in the formation of numerous oleoresin ducts that ooze benzoin. Used since ancient times and traded in Asia for the last three thousand years, benzoin has always been a major commodity of the luxury trade and is widely used in folk medicine.

The resin pieces look and feel like misshapen and hollow gold coins, light in the hand. This sense of lightweight porousness and softness is reflected in the light, flat nature of the aroma. The scent is predominantly soft vanilla, due to the presence of the aroma molecule vanillin. The soft, sweet, warm body note evolves into a balsamic, powdery finish.

Available as an absolute

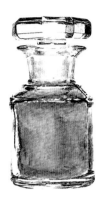

Bushman's Candle

Sarcocaulon mossamedense

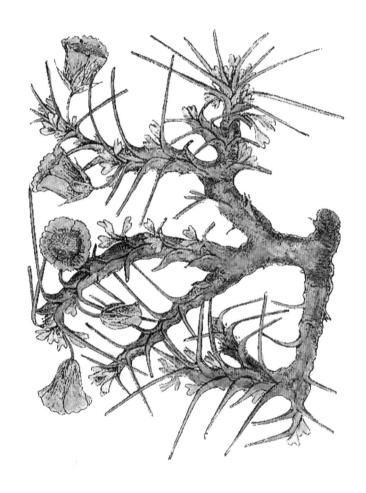

W hen this plant dies, its wood decomposes, leaving on the ground a hollow fallen bark that is gathered by the Himba tribe in Namibia. The waxy content of the bark makes it burnable as candles or kindling, yielding a musky and spicy smoke. The warm aroma of bushman's candle is filled with notes of caramel, vanilla, and amber, making it well suited for adding a resinous facet to florals.

Available as a resinoid

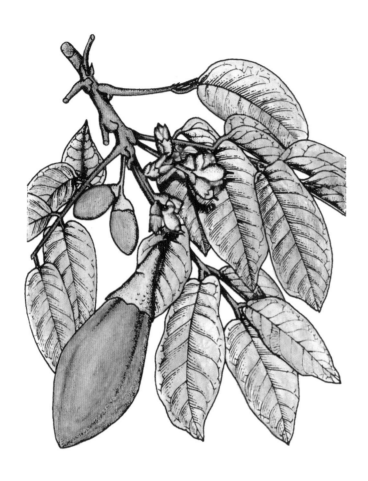

Elemi

Canarium luzonicum

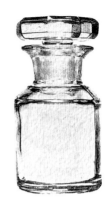

The name *elemi* is from an Arabic phrase meaning "above and below"—an abbreviation of the alchemical maxim "as above, so below," which speaks of elemi's effect on the emotional and spiritual planes. When fresh, the fragrant soft white resin has a honey-like consistency, but with age it gets harder and yellower. The essential oil, distilled from the resin, is fresh, bright, and lemony. From the same family as frankincense, it smells somewhat like it, but lighter, greener, and more peppery.

Available as an essential oil

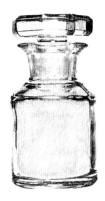

Frankin-cense

Various *Boswellia* species (*sacra* or *carteri*, *neglecta*, *frereana*)

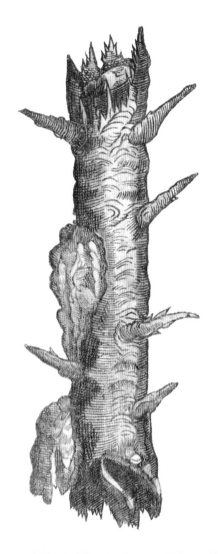

The name *frankincense* is derived from an Old French phrase meaning "choice incense." In the regions of the Arabian Peninsula and the Horn of Africa that grow frankincense, it is still deeply woven into medicinal practice and religious and social rituals. It is used to flavor coffee and to treat dental problems, arthritis, and coughs. It is also believed to promote peace and harmony, and therefore is burned at weddings and religious celebrations.

Frankincense was used for embalming in ancient Egypt, and the resin was considered divine. The method of collection is unchanged since ancient times: incisions are made into the bark of the small trees, and the resin oozes out, hardens, and is scraped off. The resin pieces look like chrysoberyl jewels in the hand, all irregular shapes. When you hold them, the delicious green apple, resinous, and lemony scent rubs off and makes you feel anointed. One of the main components of frankincense resin is boswellic acid, which is anti-cancerous and anti-inflammatory.

Available as an essential oil and as an absolute

The gum is procured by making longitudinal incisions through the bark in the months of May and December. . . . The operation is simple, and requires no skill on the part of the operator. On its first appearance the gum comes forth white as milk, and according to its degree of fluidity, finds its way to the ground, or concretes on the branch near the place from which it first issued, from whence it is collected by men and boys employed to look after the trees by the different families who possess the land in which they grow.

—Flückiger and Hanbury, *Pharmacographia*, 1879

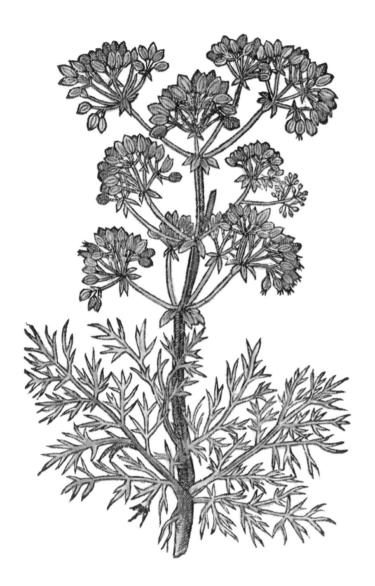

Galbanum

Ferula galbaniflua
(or *Ferula gummosa*)

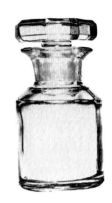

Galbanum has a powerfully intense aroma: sharply green, spicy, leaf-like, with notes of green bell peppers. The plant oozes a milky juice from the lower part of the stems and the roots; the stem is cut, and the resin is collected after it hardens into small tears. Galbanum has a long history of being used in medicine (it is antimicrobial), incense, and flavoring. It is mentioned in the original recipe in the Bible for the holy incense: "And the Lord said unto Moses, Take unto thee sweet spices, stacte, and onycha, and galbanum; these sweet spices with pure frankincense: of each there shall be a like weight" (Exodus 30:34).

Available as an essential oil

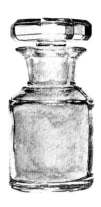

Labdanum

Cistus ladanifer

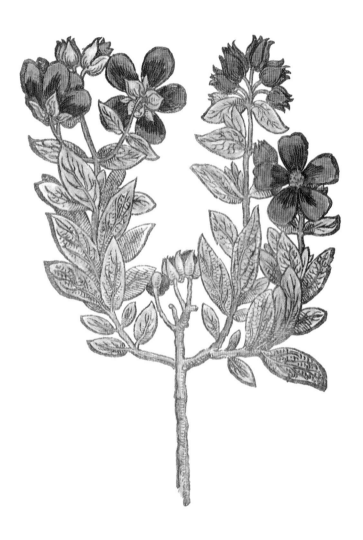

Labdanum is the resinous exudation of the leaves and twigs of the rockrose plant, whose flower looks like a single-petaled flat rose. The sticky, ambery resin droplets are found in the twigs and on the underside of the leaves. The twigs are boiled, and the resin comes to the surface and is skimmed off. Labdanum has a pronounced sweet, balsamic, rich ambery odor, with animalic undertones. This unique aroma is the natural foundational essence in all amber perfumes.

Available as an absolute

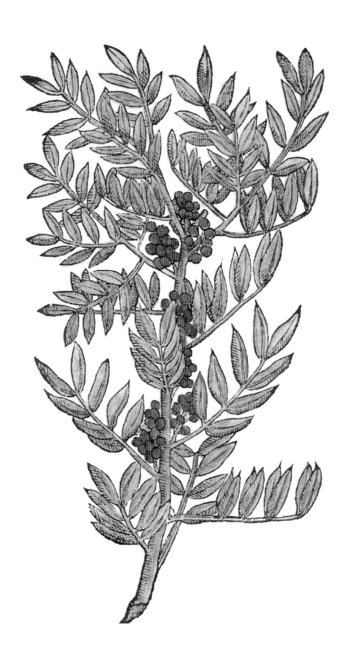

Mastic

Pistacia lentiscus

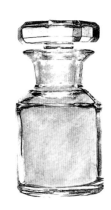

Mastic is traditionally from the Greek island of Chios. Incisions made into the trunk of this small tree exude a resin that hardens and becomes brittle. The best mastic comes in pale yellow, pear-shaped tears, and has a fresh balsamic, penetrating leafy aroma. The English word *masticate* comes from the Latin *masticare*, meaning "to chew," which is in turn from the Greek *mastikhan*, "to grind the teeth." The name *mastic* derives from the same Greek word, and mastic resin was used to make the original chewing gum. The taste is mild and resinous. When chewed, it becomes soft like chewing gum and sweetens the breath.

Available as an essential oil

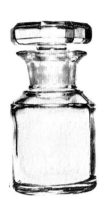

Myrrh

Commiphora myrrha

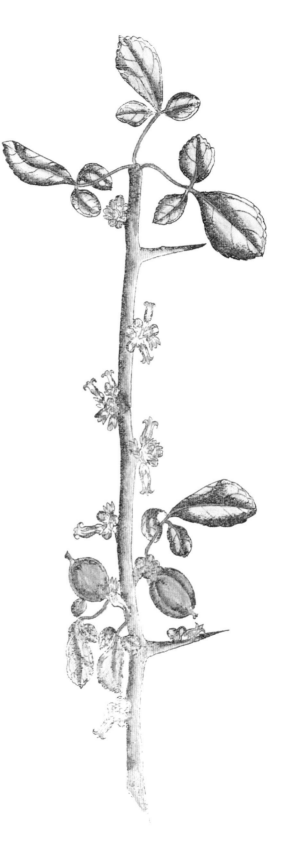

Myrrh is always mentioned alongside frankincense as one of the two rock stars of the ancient incense realm. Whereas frankincense is pale and sweet, myrrh is dark and bitter (and gets darker with age). In fact, the word *murr* in Arabic means "bitter." In the long-ago past, myrrh's beautifully scented incense smoke was offered up to the gods as a substitute for human and animal sacrifice. Myrrh's warm, balsamic, sweet, and spicy aroma was also used to disguise bad smells. It was used by many ancient peoples for anointing, and some resin in King Tutankhamen's tomb was still fragrant when found. And it was used to embalm the body of Jesus Christ!

Commiphora wildii, or omumbiri, a special species of myrrh collected by women in Namibia, is uplifting and relaxing, with a buttery smoothness. The aroma is fresh but warm, with hints of lemon, evolving into a sweet balsamic drydown.

Both myrrhs are available as essential oils.

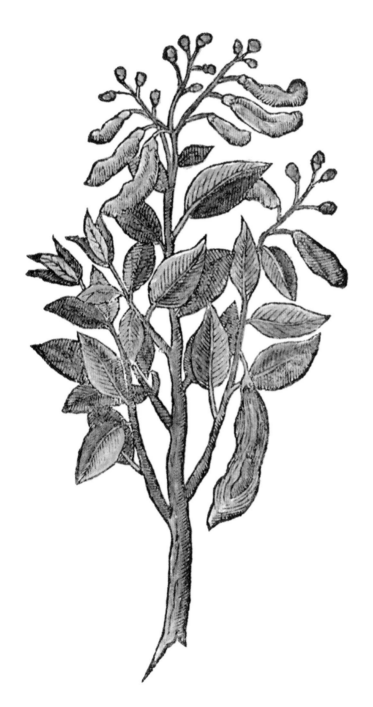

Peru Balsam

Myroxylon pereirae
(or *Myroxylon balsamum*
var. *pereirae*)

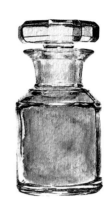

The scientific name of Peru balsam is from the Greek words *myron*, meaning "sweet oil" or "perfume," and *xylon*, meaning "wood." This fragrant resin smells like cinnamon when fresh, but more like vanilla as it ages! The tree doesn't exude the resin naturally, but requires unusually heavy tapping. The trunk must be beaten, stripped of its bark, covered with a cloth, and scorched with a torch to release the flow of resin. The saturated cloth is then boiled and pressed to separate the resin. Even though it endures this intense harvesting process, the tree can live for centuries. The aroma is thick, rich, sweet, dessert-y. Ironically, the resin has many uses for wound healing!

Available as a resin

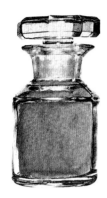

Poplar Buds

Populus ×jackii, balsamifera, and other species

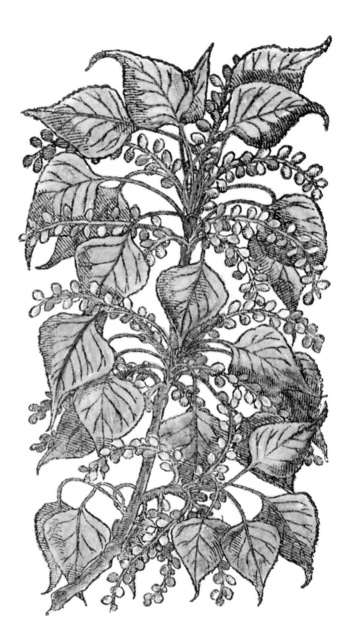

The resin that comes from poplar buds is commonly called Balm of Gilead, after the perfume mentioned in the Old Testament. Poplar buds, however, are a product of the New World—in fact, Native Americans used their resin medicinally, to make salves for wounds and rashes as well as pain and soreness. Poplar buds have a very complex and tenacious but sweet balsamic aroma, which contains notes of apricots, cinnamon, and osmanthus, as well as sweet balsam, precious wood, and leather. The winter buds contain the fragrant resin, which coats the young leaves when they unfurl from the bud.

Available as an absolute

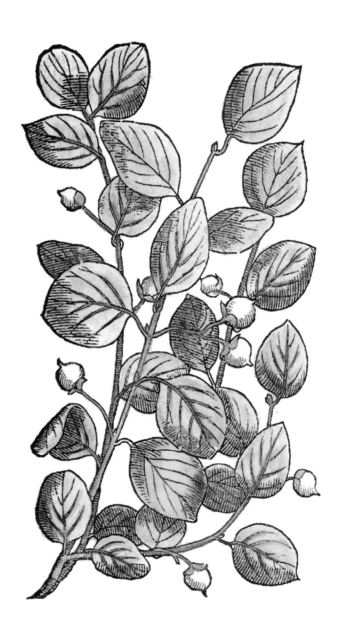

Styrax

Liquidambar orientalis

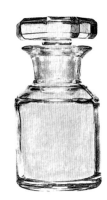

Styrax, also called storax, oozes from incisions made in the trunk of the tree and congeals into tears on exposure to the air. The balsamic, dry, sweet floral scent is reminiscent of hyacinth and lilacs, with a touch of cinnamon. There are also traces of styrene—which smells like airplane glue!

Available as an essential oil

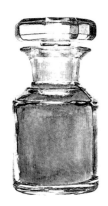

Tolu Balsam

Myroxylon balsamum
(or *Myroxylon balsamum*
var. *balsamum*)

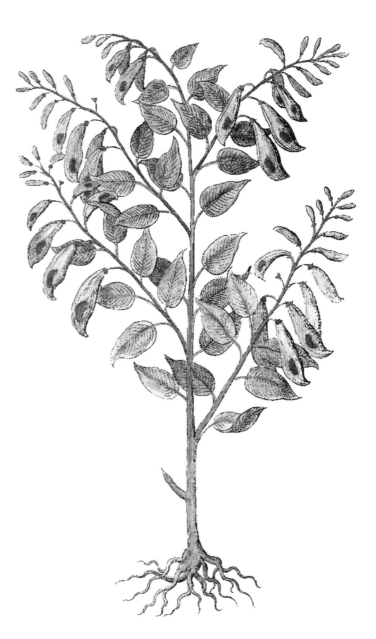

Like a number of other resins, the brown, syrupy Tolu balsam is produced by making incisions in the bark of the tree. The sweet, rich aroma is a beautiful blend of vanilla and cinnamon with delicate hyacinth facets—it blends well with any other essence. Tolu is closely related to Peru balsam; while Peru is spicier, tolu is more floral.

Available as an absolute

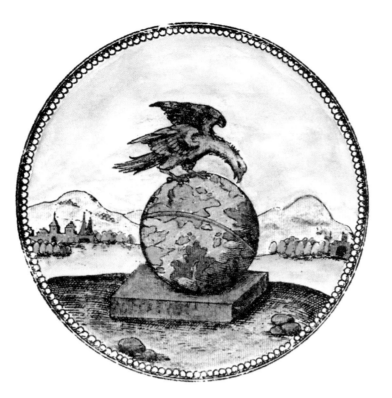

14
Symbolorum
et
Emblematum

The *Symbolorum et Emblematum* was the first natural history emblem book, and one of the first books to use engraved intaglio plates for natural history illustrations. The book consists of four "centuries" of one hundred entries each, devoted to plants, quadrupeds (real and fantastic), birds, and fish. The German scholar Joachim Camerarius published the first three centuries separately between 1590 and 1596, and his son Ludwig Camerarius added the century of fish in 1604. There were a number of subsequent editions collecting all four centuries in a single volume, and the edition of 1654 is in the collection of the Aftel Archive of Curious Scents.

Each entry consists of four parts: a motto, the emblem itself (that is, an allegorical illustration), a verse epigram, and a prose commentary that offers an entertaining and imaginative amalgam of zoology, botany, and moral wisdom. The emblems are meticulously rendered as copperplate engravings and set off in jewel-like circular frames. Their style blends the close observation of nature with mythical archetypes. Precious and exquisite, these visually arresting images function like a dream world that you can enter on any page.

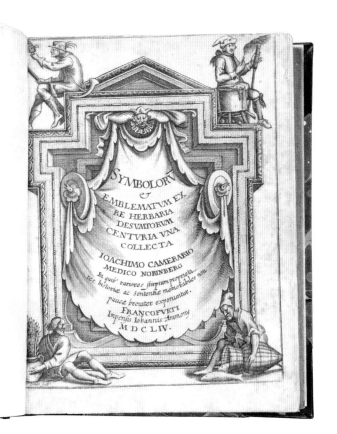

LEFT

The title page of the Aftel Archive's 1654 edition of the Symbolorum et Emblematum.

BELOW

An entry from the Symbolorum. *On the right-hand page is a motto ("If you don't break, you cannot be"), an emblem, and a verse epigram ("Lofty wisdom is girded round with worries, but it also overflows with sweet delights"). On the left-hand page is a learned commentary full of allusions to classical authors.*

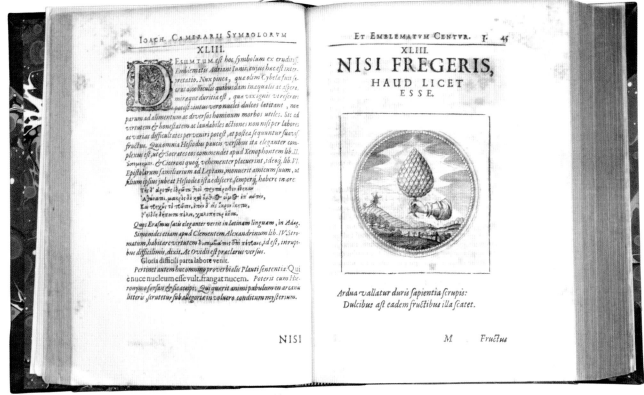

Like Aesop, Camerarius anthropomorphized his animals to show that we can learn from nature. The mackerel display unintelligent behavior by wanting to join their friends in a wicker-basket trap. In contrast, the parrotfish perceive the danger and are pulling on their friends' tails to free them.

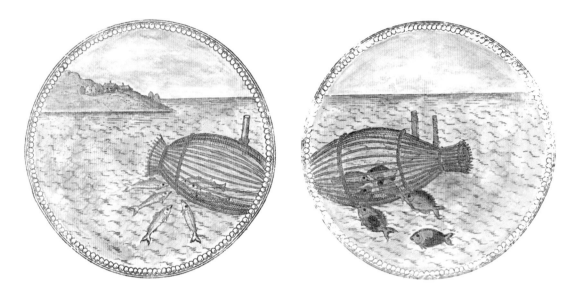

The epigram for the dumb mackerel reads: "These want to go in, but those [inside] want to break out of the trap; many are equally stupid as the mackerel."

Whereas for the parrotfish, the epigram reads: "Good fortune calls for loyalty, but adversity demands it."

Sometimes Camerarius focused on rarities: for example, he included a musk deer and a four-headed hydra. In this way he expressed his admiration of the miraculous power of nature and its surprising, and sometimes hidden, intelligence.

The elephant had great importance for Camerarius, not only because it is the biggest land animal, but because he believed (per Pliny) that the elephant possessed a humanlike intelligence and spiritual life. One emblem depicts the elephant's alleged habit of walking to a particular river to purify itself and worship the moon.

The Great Seal of the United States, the world's best-known coat of arms, owes a great debt to Camerarius's emblem of an eagle. The *Symbolorum et Emblematum* was a favorite of Benjamin Franklin, who owned a 1702 edition and drew inspiration from it for his designs for the first American coins and banknotes. In 1776, Charles Thomson (1729–1824), a classical scholar and Secretary of the Continental Congress, designed the Great Seal. His main source was the heraldic eagle emblem in Benjamin Franklin's copy of Camerarius's book, which shows an olive branch near its right talon, and a bundle of flaming arrows near its left.

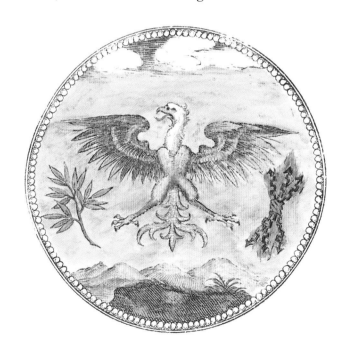

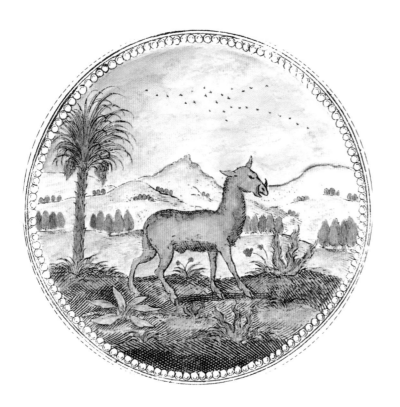

15
Musk

[Musk] masters and drives out bad vapors and kills demons and spirits. . . . If used over a long period of time it gets rid of evil.

—Ancient Chinese source quoted in Anya H. King, *Scent from the Garden of Paradise: Musk and the Medieval Islamic World,* 2017

OPPOSITE

The musk deer exhibit at the Aftel Archive, featuring a papier-mâché musk deer by Erin Cramer, 2015.

In the glass box are Tonquin musk grains from 1906 in the original bottle.

On the tray, from left to right, are musk bottled by I. D. Edrehi, Tonquin musk bottled by Rich's; Tonquin musk bottled by Fritzsche Brothers, and Tonquin musk grains bottled by Fritzsche Brothers. All are about a century old.

Musk has been used almost as long as there has been civilization itself. The musk deer (*Moschus moschiferus*) produces one of the most historically significant and mysterious scent ingredients. The male deer's musk pouch is filled with irregularly shaped black grains, which develop the characteristic scent as they dry. Strange, beautiful, uncategorizable, and feral, the aroma pushes you out of your comfort zone without pushing you away—you are still drawn in.

The power of musk as an aphrodisiac is legendary. The smell of authentic musk is erotic, reminiscent of sweat and the hairy regions of the human body. The aroma has nothing in common with modern synthetic musk, which is used in everything from fine fragrance to laundry dryer strips. Natural musk is no longer used in the commercial perfume industry, and the animal has been endangered for years.

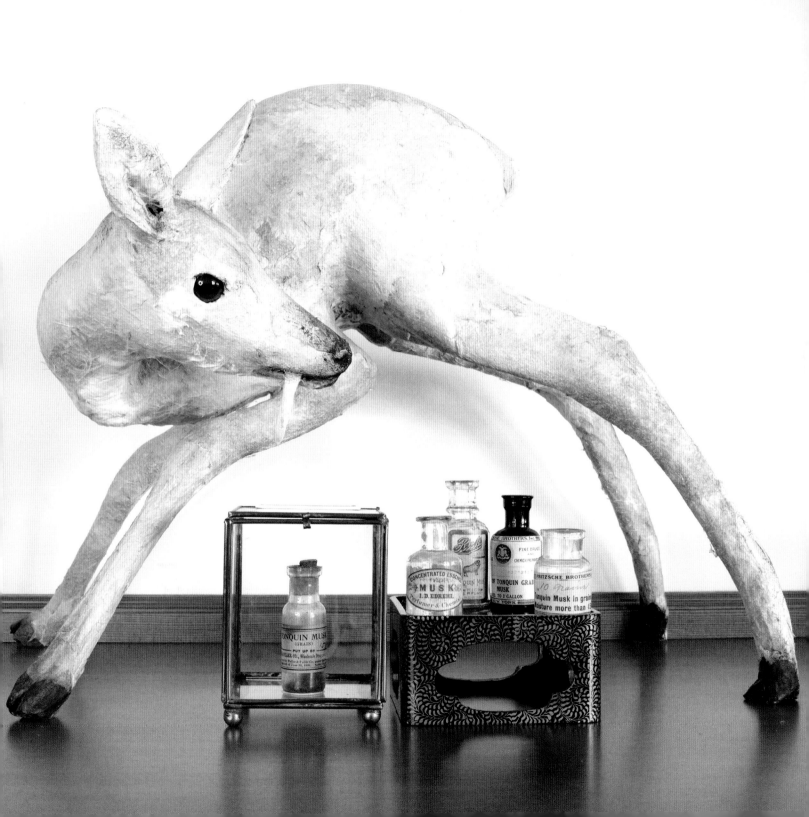

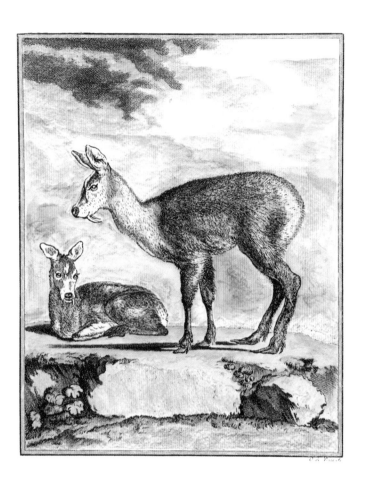

At Szuchuan the musk is already subject to frequent adulterations. In order to detect these, certain definite methods are employed there. If the odour is not satisfactory, or if other doubts exist as to the genuine character, a small incision is made in the musk-bag, a sample taken out, and thrown in water. If the sample remains crumbly, the musk is genuine, but if it dissolves, it is adulterated. Or a sample is placed on a glowing piece of charcoal; if it melts and swells up, the musk is good; if it suddenly becomes hard, it must be regarded as adulterated.

—Schimmel & Co., April 1906, p. 94

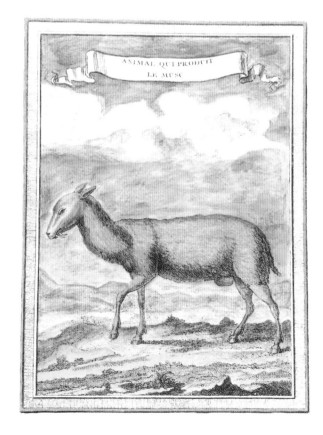

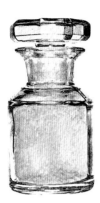

Ambrette

Abelmoschus moschatus

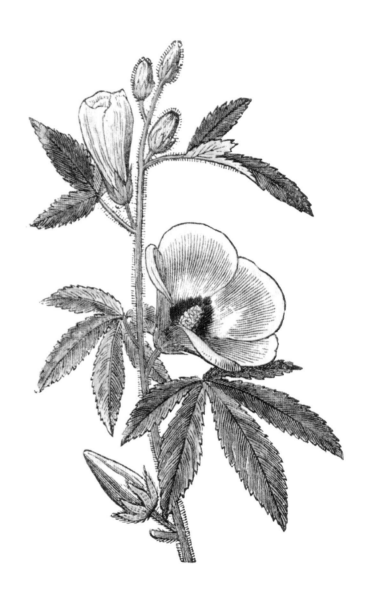

Ambrette seed, from the hibiscus plant, is known as the botanical equivalent of musk. Ambrette seed oil is smooth, rich, sweet, floral, and musky all at once, like brandy or overripe fruit. Incredibly tenacious and long-lasting, ambrette has the uncanny ability to enhance florals. The absolute is the finest version to use in a perfume, making it longer-lasting, enhancing the other essences, and bottom-feeding the overall aroma with clean, musky notes.

Available as a CO_2 extract and an absolute

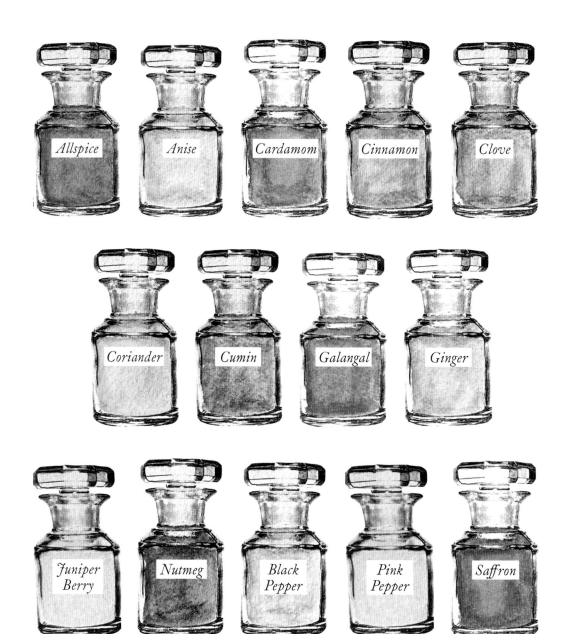

Allspice Anise Cardamom Cinnamon Clove

Coriander Cumin Galangal Ginger

Juniper Berry Nutmeg Black Pepper Pink Pepper Saffron

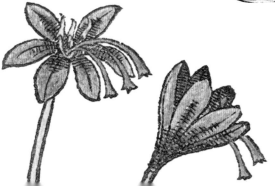

16
The Spice Family

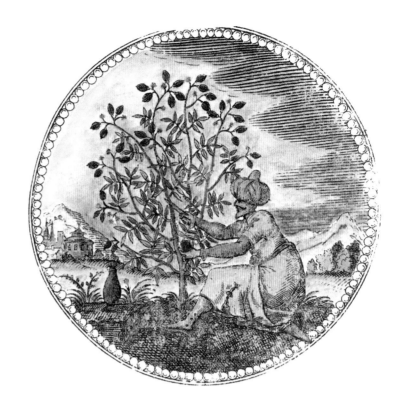

Spices come from seeds, roots, and bark—often from plants grown in faraway places, giving them their tinge of the exotic. From time immemorial, spices have inspired and encouraged the art of the perfumer. People have an innate love for their aromas, which are ancient, dusted with history from distant lands, rich and intense, but also comforting and familiar. Civilizations were built, and fortunes made and lost, in pursuit of precious spices. The Sumerian word for "perfume" is made up of the cuneiform signs representing "oil" and "sweet." In that early period, as for millennia afterward, oils were infused with spices to create perfumes.

Spices are the richest and most intense family of scents; in a perfume they vivify neighboring essences, not only introducing new aromas to the blend but also highlighting those that are already present. They offer the greatest potential for creating contrast in a perfume. In comparison to the attractive aromas of flowers, for example, spice aromas generally evolved as a deterrent to predators, and indeed are sometimes toxic to them. Yet the same spicy smells that repel pests also attract humans to use them in flavor and fragrance.

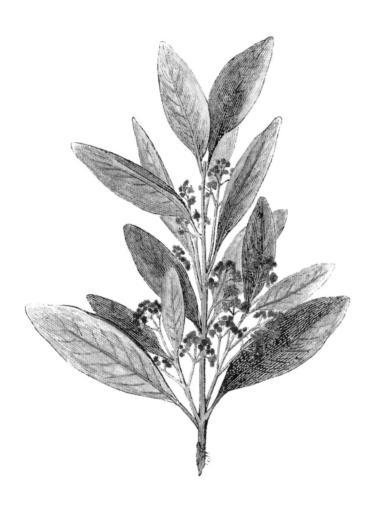

Allspice

Pimenta dioica

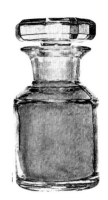

Allspice, also called pimento berry, smells like a composite of cloves, cinnamon, and nutmeg—hence its common name. The aroma is sweet, warm, and woody, with tea-like facets and a round aromatic shape. The dominant aroma molecule in allspice is eugenol, which smells like clove, but allspice's floral components soften and sweeten it. Allspice is useful in creating fragrances as an agreeable and indeterminate softer spice that blends with almost any other essence and is not overly culinary.

Available as a CO_2 extract and an essential oil. The essential oil is sharper than the CO_2.

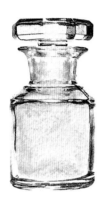

Anise

Pimpinella anisum

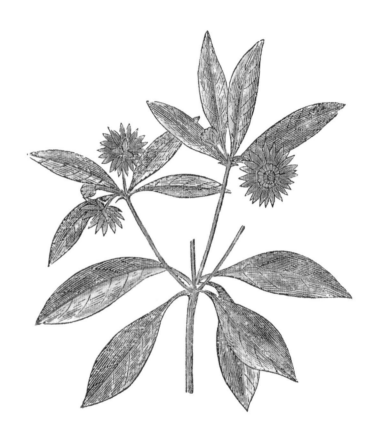

Anise was one of the spices most valued by the ancients for remedies and has been used since 1500 BC. It was said that suspending the plant near one's pillow to smell while asleep would keep away bad dreams. The aroma is clean and licorice-y, with a sweet, warm, and fruity character and a refreshing camphor facet. Its character is determined primarily by the molecule anethole.

Available as a CO_2 extract and an essential oil. The CO_2, derived from star anise, smells like licorice candy and childhood, and is the finest.

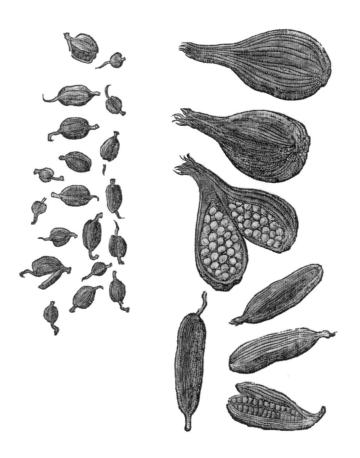

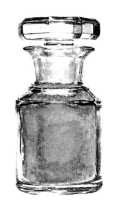

Cardamom

Elettaria cardamomum

Cardamom is the third most expensive spice in the world, after saffron and vanilla. The fruit, densely packed with seeds, is harvested while still firm and unripe, and then dried. The major chemical components of the scent are cineol (camphor) and pinene (pine), giving it a full-bodied, high-intensity aroma. Each form of extraction yields a slightly different-smelling essence, and emphasizes the different facets of cardamom: warm, camphoraceous, bittersweet, fresh, spicy, and floral, with facets of mint, eucalyptus, and black pepper.

Available as an essential oil, CO_2 extract, and absolute. The essential oil is the sharpest and most aggressive, the CO_2 is warmer and softer, and the absolute is the most multilayered—round and warm, without any scent of eucalyptus.

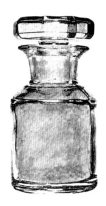

Cinnamon

Cinnamomum zeylanicum
(or *Cinnamomum verum*)

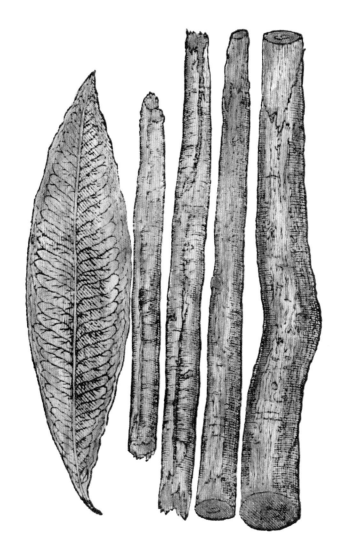

Cinnamon was once the king of spices, and its current status, largely limited to desserts, deserves to be reconsidered. It was first used in China around 2500 BC for medicinal purposes. People often confuse cinnamon and cassia, which are closely related plants but have different aromatic facets: cassia has coarser and thicker bark and shares with cinnamon a sweet, spicy aroma, but with more pungent and harsh bitter aspects. Cinnamon is sharply aromatic, warm, sweet, and dry, with more delicate facets. Cinnamon possesses a note of clove from a small amount of eugenol, which is not present in cassia.

The best-quality cinnamon oil opens with a candylike freshness, evolves into a tenacious aroma that is equally sweet and spicy, and finishes off with a dry sweetness that is irresistibly tied to baked goods.

Available as an essential oil and a CO_2 extract

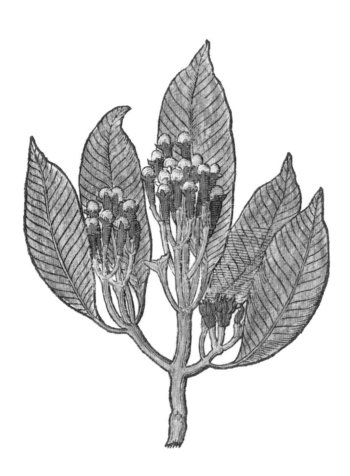

Clove

Syzygium aromaticum

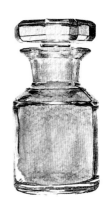

Cloves—whose name comes from the Latin *clavus*, "nail," because of their nail-like shape—are the unopened buds of the tree. After the closed buds are picked, they are dried in the sun, and their color changes from rose to dark reddish brown. Their scent is largely made up of the molecule eugenol, and it has a pointed and strong aromatic intensity, with both peppery camphor facets and floral, carnation-like ones. Clove—the most floral of all the spices—has historically been blended with rose to create a carnation fragrance.

Available as an essential oil and an absolute. My favorite is the warm, rich, round absolute, which has none of the medicinal facets of the essential oil.

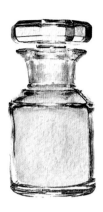

Coriander

Coriandrum sativum

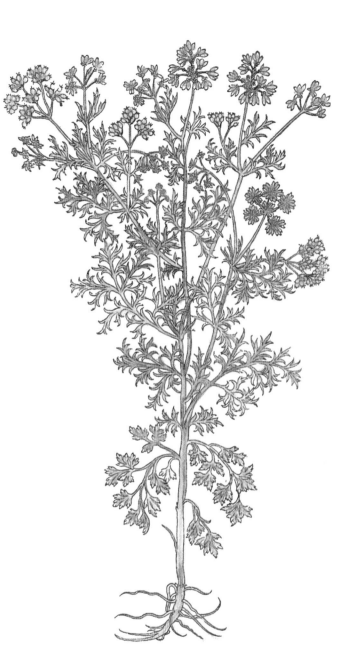

The name *coriander* comes from the Greek word *koris*, meaning "bedbug," because of the "buggy" odor of the unripe seeds. Coriander has floral facets from a large amount of linalool, along with the rosy molecules geraniol and geranyl acetate. The aroma of coriander seeds is sweet, woody, and spicy, while the polarizing aroma of the leaves is pungent, soapy, and herbal. Coriander is useful as a green, floral top note—a rarity in the natural perfumer's palette.

Available as an essential oil and a CO_2 extract

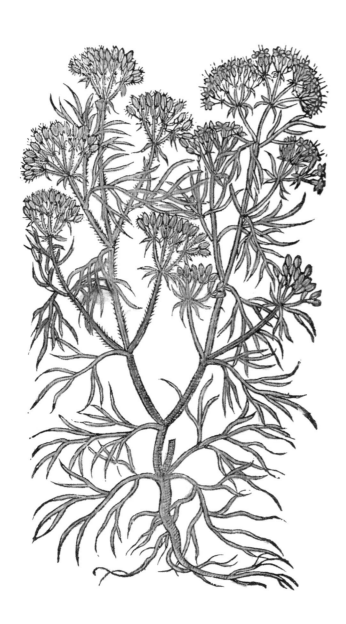

Cumin

Cuminum cyminum

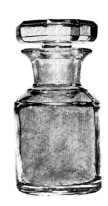

Cumin, a small, gray-green seed, was called *sughandan* in Sanskrit, meaning "good smelling." Ancient Egyptians used it to mummify royalty. Powerfully dense and heavy, cumin has high odor and flavor intensity, with complex facets that can lead it in many directions: nutty, earthy, spicy, fatty, and penetrating.

It is used in perfume in tiny quantities to add a human ("sweaty") note to compositions.

Available as an essential oil and a CO_2 extract. The difference between the two is amazing. The CO_2 is fresh and bright: complex, spicy, and nutty—and reminiscent of the human body. The essential oil is acrid, vegetal, musty, slightly putrid, and sweaty.

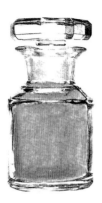

Galangal

Alpinia galanga

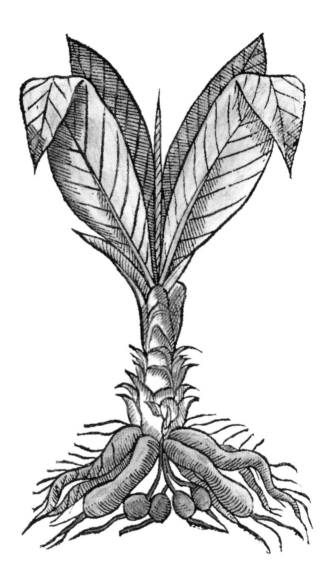

Distilled from the roots, galangal essential oil smells like a mixture of cardamom, ginger, and saffron. Its fresh, peppery warmth includes a dash of coolness. Complex and tangy, it has the ability to enhance other spices. Plutarch noted that Egyptians burned galangal to disinfect the air.

Available as an essential oil

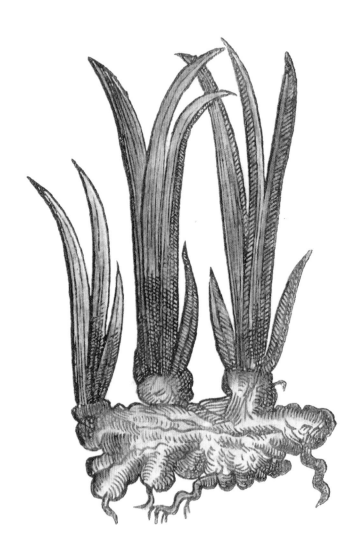

Ginger

Zingiber officinale

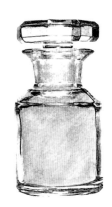

The name *ginger* comes from the Sanskrit *shringavera*, meaning "shaped like a deer's antlers." Fresh ginger is more aromatic than dried. When fresh, its character is spicy, refreshing, sweet, and delicate. The presence of the aroma molecule citral gives it a lemon-like facet. The essential oil carries the distinctive aroma of ginger from the predominant volatile molecule zingiberene—which makes up about 70 percent of the essence when extracted from the fresh root. Ginger root's characteristic pungency comes from heavier molecules like gingerol, which are not volatile and therefore get left behind when the essential oil is distilled from the plant. Fresh ginger essential oil is lemon-like and delicate, unlike dried ginger essential oil, which is heavy and musty.

Available as essential oils from both dried and fresh ginger

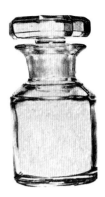

Juniper Berry

Juniperus communis

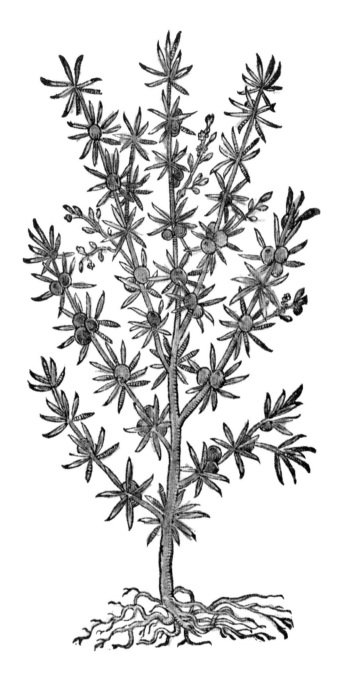

In ancient times, the berries, root, and bark of juniper were used for medicinal purposes and to keep away evil spirits. When people think of the aroma of juniper, they think of gin, because juniper is what gives gin its characteristic flavor and aroma. Juniper's berrylike fruits contain sacs of flavorful oils; they take two years to ripen, turning from green to blue. The essential oil from the ripe berries smells sweet but tastes bitter. It adds a dry sparkle to the opening of a perfume, along with warm balsamic, coniferous undertones. It contains the aroma molecules geraniol (light rosy) and limonene (citrus).

Available as an essential oil

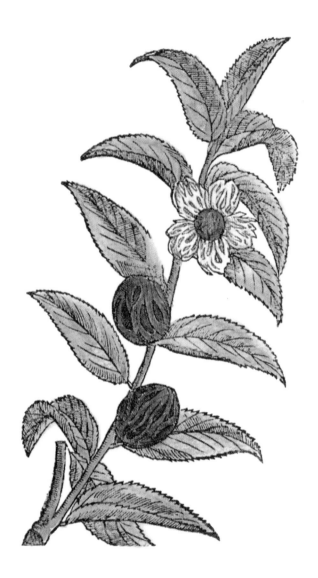

Nutmeg

Myristica fragrans

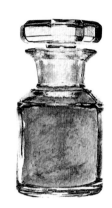

Nutmeg is a light brown, ovoid, wrinkled dried seed inside a blackish brown nut. The nut is dried in the sun until the inner seed rattles when shaken. The name comes from the Latin *nux muscatus*, meaning "musky nut," after its musky sweetness. Nutmeg combines the sweetness of spice with the warmth of wood in just the right proportions, which made it an important component in the original formula for Coca-Cola. Nutmeg has a rounded and powdery aromatic shape and medium to light intensity. It is especially useful in shading florals in a perfume, adding a triumvirate of warmth, wood, and spice facets in a single essence.

Available as an essential oil and an absolute

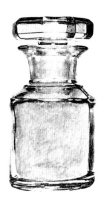

Black Pepper

Piper nigrum

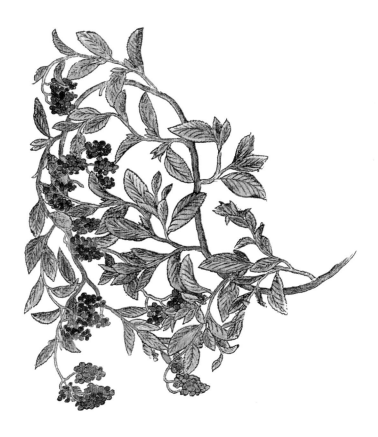

Black pepper is the most important table spice in the world. The globular, wrinkled peppercorns are actually dried fruits. The essential oil's aroma—clean, dry, woody, and penetrating—is both familiar and utterly new. There is a subtle floral facet to the aroma due to the molecule linalool. Using the essential oil for flavor is a revelation, because it has all the taste but none of the heat. The molecule responsible for the pungency—piperine—is too heavy to be extracted in the distillation process. In a perfume, black pepper essential oil brings focus and shape to the opening, blending well with most other essences.

Available as an essential oil

The general prevalence during the middle ages of *pepper-rents*, which consisted in an obligation imposed upon a tenant to supply his lord with a certain quantity of pepper, generally a pound, at stated times, shows how acceptable was this favourite condiment, and how great the desire of the wealthier classes to secure a supply of it when the market was not always certain.

—Flückiger and Hanbury,
Pharmacographia, 1879

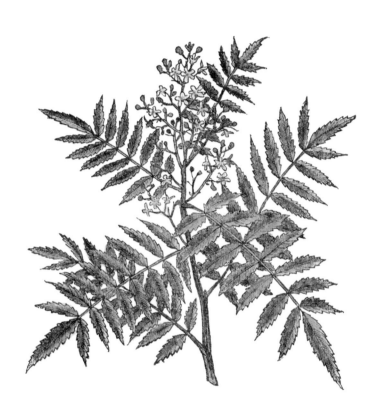

Pink Pepper

Schinus molle

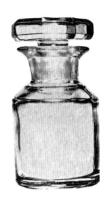

Pink pepper is not a true pepper, but a member of the cashew family. Its round, pepper-like shape and size contribute to the confusion. Pink pepper has top notes similar to black pepper, but they are combined with fruitier and creamier components. It is distinguished by its dry berry facets that bring a clean freshness, punctuated with spice. Pink pepper essential oil is welcome in any blend, with its clear pine and mild floral facets.

Available as an essential oil

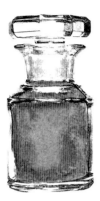

Saffron

Crocus sativus

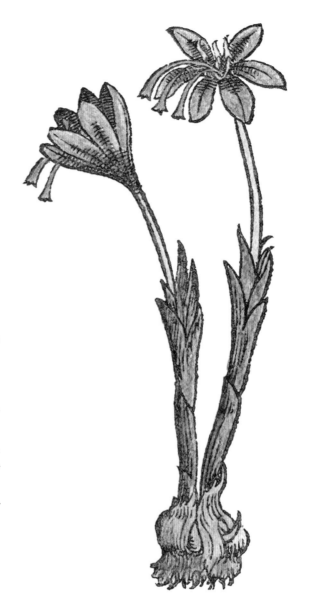

The dried stigmata of the saffron flower—long, orange-red filaments—have long been highly prized for cooking, medicine, dyeing, and perfume. The many uses of saffron illustrate how, in the past, these pursuits were knitted together in a more holistic fashion. Saffron offers a multisensory experience: its aroma is almost impossible to separate from its taste and color. Although it's a spice, it doesn't have any of the sharpness typical of spices; instead, its aroma is flat, deep, and heavy, with an earthiness. It's useful as a top note, lending an earthy denseness to neighboring top notes that are too sharp.

Available as an absolute

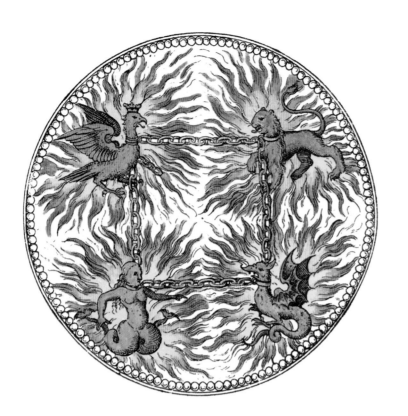

17
Cabinet of Curiosities

Wardrobes with their shelves, desks with their drawers, and chests with their false bottoms are veritable organs of the secret psychological life.
—Bachelard

The cabinet of curiosities or *Wunderkammer* (literally "chamber of wonders") was the forerunner of our natural history museum, and the first cabinets of curiosities were in fact whole rooms where people displayed extraordinary and bizarre objects they collected from all over the world. Later "cabinet of curiosities" came to mean a piece of furniture in which such a collection was displayed. It was a miniature museum whose many drawers, compartments, and shelves brimmed with natural wonders: bezoar stones, shells, skeletons of strange animals, miniature laboratory glassware, bottles of unguents, hunks of ambergris, taxidermied specimens, musk pods.

The Aftel Archive's cabinet of curiosities contains the strange, the rare, the botanical, the imaginative, the bizarre, and the handcrafted. Like earlier cabinets, it is designed to fill you with wonder and surprise, stop your forward motion, and drop you into a contemplative state of wonder at our curious aromatic world. Our tiger oak cabinet from the 1850s has curved glass doors and glass sides so you can see the curiosities in the round when you're standing in front of it.

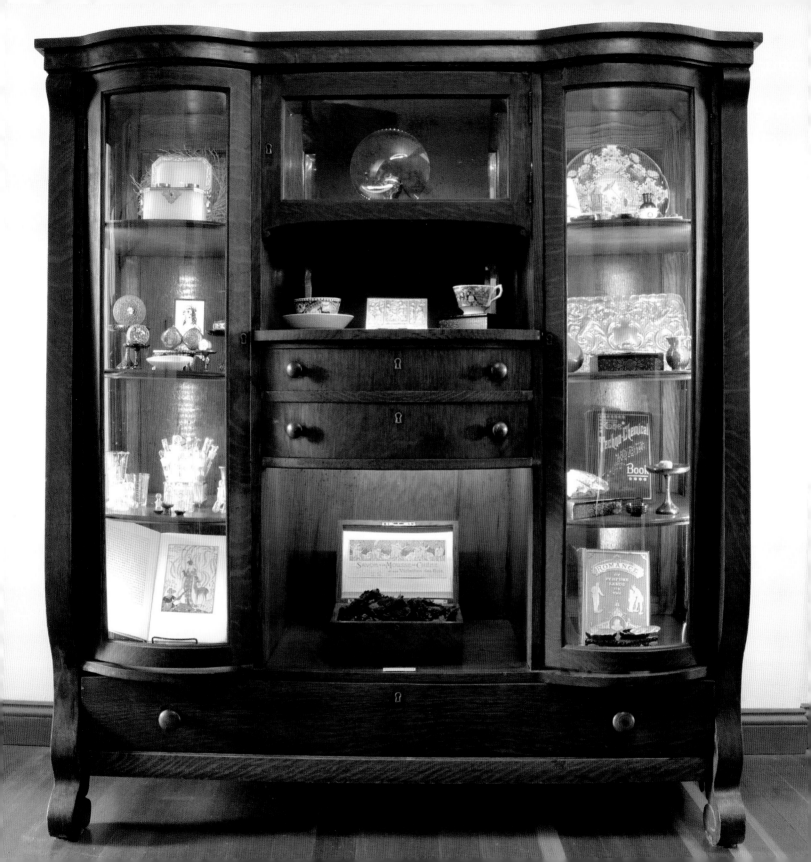

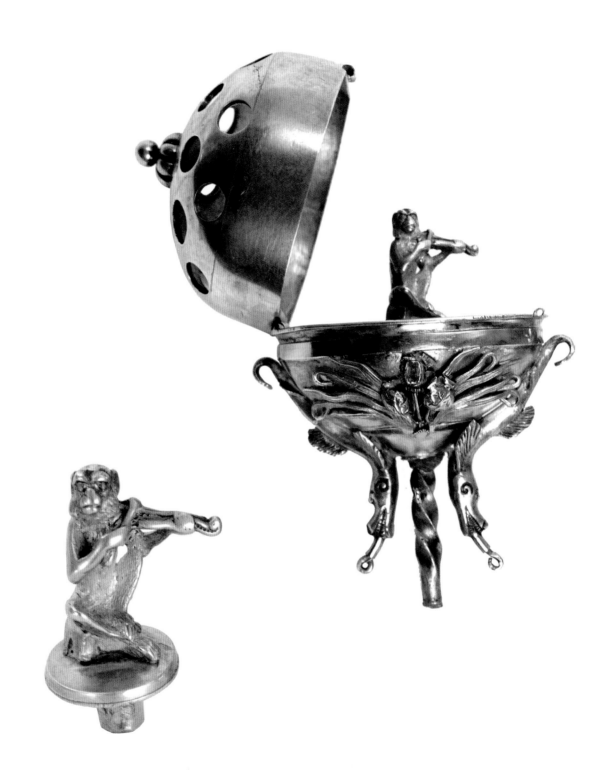

Rare Museum-Quality French Pomander, circa 1790

Pomanders (from the French *pomme d'ambre*, "apple of amber") were open metalwork balls made to hold aromatic spices, herbs, and even ambergris (hence the name)—to ward off every kind of plague, pestilence, and bad smell of the day. The crown jewel in our cabinet of curiosities—quite literally—is our rare and unique artisan-made pomander from the late 1700s. Worn around a French aristocrat's wrist or neck, this superb pomander would have brought relief to the senses when lifted to the nose. Its pierced dome of sterling silver in the shape of an egg would have held a piece of fabric wadding doused with scent. In the lower section, the arched necks of a pair of serpents are twined around a gold stem. The sides are adorned with a solid gold poppy head, a cut ruby, and a turquoise cabochon. The perfume reservoir is capped with an extraordinary stopper in the form of a monkey playing the violin. The French inscription translates as "Live, little fish [as well-wrought art], that you might live on after me [the engraver]!"

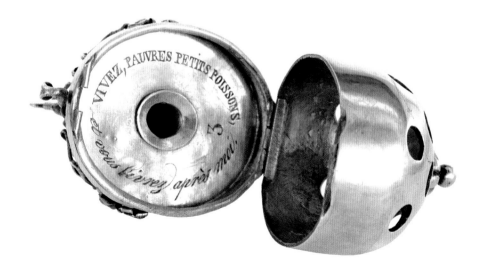

Patches and Patch Boxes

Patch boxes came into use during the eighteenth century at the court of Louis XV, where the use of beauty patches was popular. A beauty patch was made of gummed silk and pasted on the face as a beauty mark to emphasize some facial feature, usually the cheek. The patches were made in a variety of shapes: circles, stars, crescents, diamonds, etc. Patches were carried by ladies in beautifully decorated small boxes designed for the purpose, sometimes bearing a small mirror in the lid.

The display includes, at bottom, original silk taffeta patches from the 1800s in various shapes. At top is an illustration from Eugène Rimmel's *Book of Perfumes* (1868) showing how they would have been worn.

The Aftel Archive's patch boxes include this superb handmade Art Nouveau sterling silver niello example, marked by the French goldsmith Murat between 1897 and 1910. The regal gargoyle on the front is finely articulated, with shading on his wings, body, and claws as he blends in with the fanciful leaf motif framing his body. Sprigs of roses encircle the edges of the front and the back of the box; on the reverse is a beautiful portrait of the gargoyle's impressive head with his tongue extended and flowers and decorations encircling him.

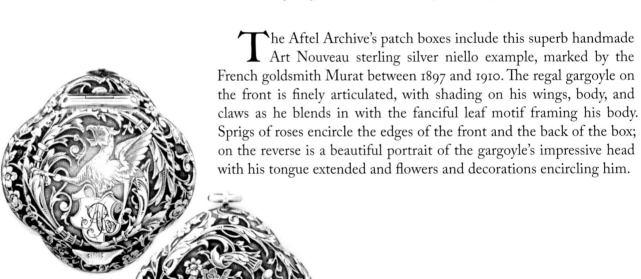

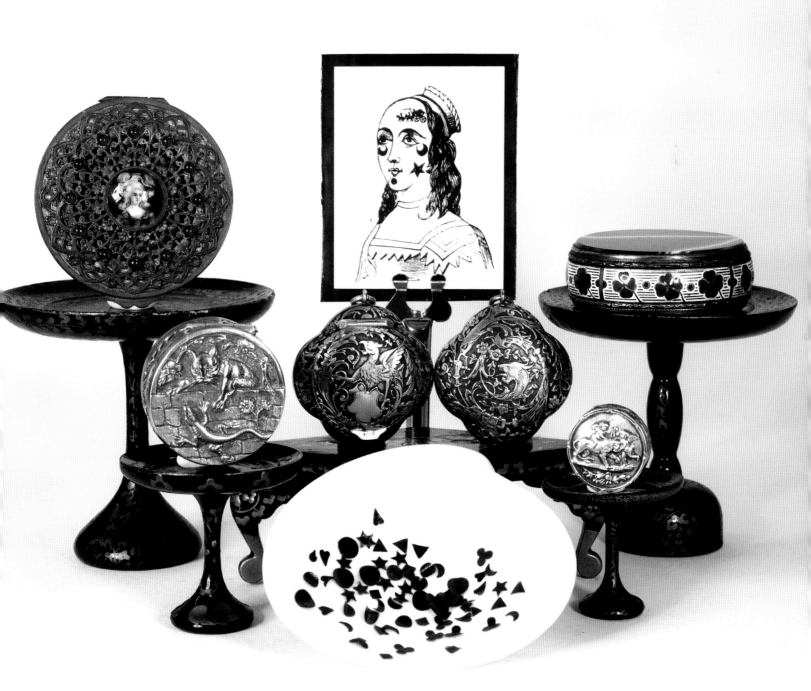

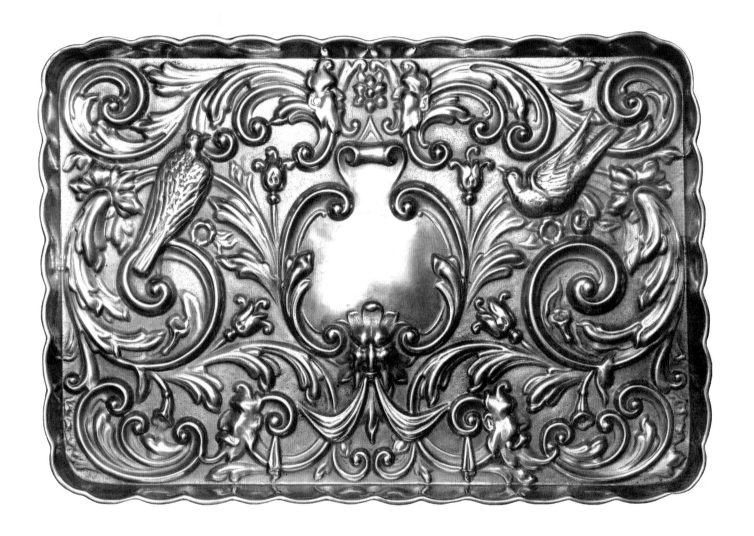

Green Man Tray

The repoussé decoration of this Art Nouveau calling-card tray features flowers, birds, and five Green Man faces! In many cultures around the world, the Green Man is a legendary being who symbolizes rebirth and the cycle of new growth in spring.

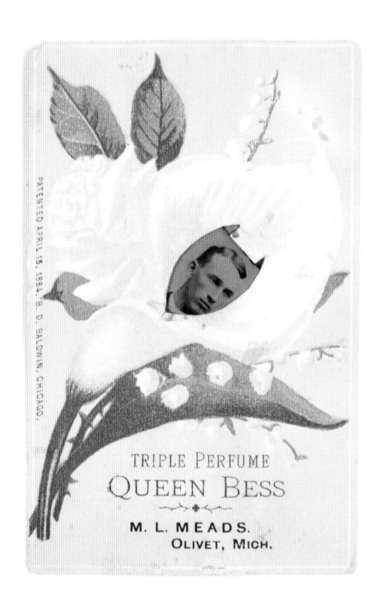

A Valentine for the Lovelorn, 1884

This love token is made from an 1884 Queen Bess perfume card. The giver cut his head out of a tintype photograph and then painstakingly embedded it in a corresponding cutout from the flower. An early instance of Photoshopping a selfie!

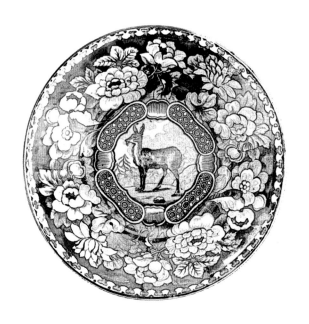

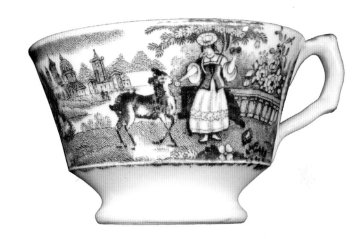

Musk Teacups and Saucer, Staffordshire, circa 1825

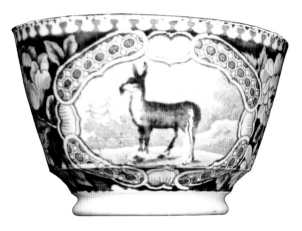

The image of the musk deer was an exotic addition to medieval bestiaries. Later it also found its way onto ceramics, along with all sorts of familiar animals—and the occasional unicorn.

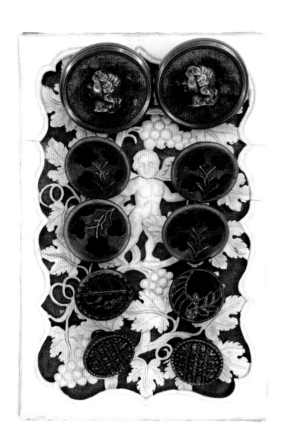

Victorian Perfume Buttons

These special buttons have an internal cavity with a piece of cloth that could be doused with fragrance. The Victorians loved fragrance, both for its help in distancing them from the miasma of the cities and for the way that it uplifted their common surroundings. They put perfume buttons like these on their clothes, and also wore pomanders or mounted them atop walking sticks.

Lalique Bronze Plaque for Parfums Fontanis, Paris, 1925

The three panels depict two women dressed in robes going through the stages of perfume production: gathering flowers, pressing and extracting the fragrance, and storing the essences. The plaque was made by the famous House of Lalique, with gold finish and a hinged easel stand.

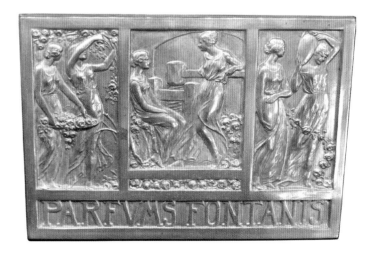

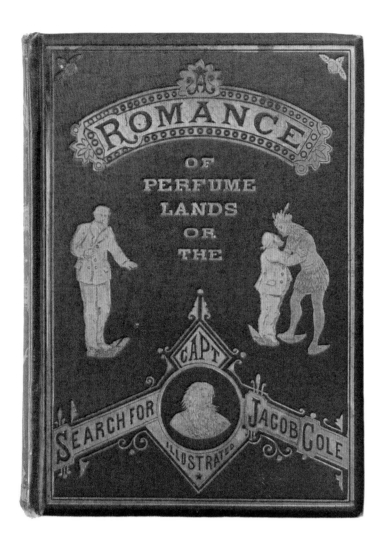

F. S. Clifford, *Romance of Perfume Lands*, 1881

This book was meant to be treasured, as you can tell from the metallic stamping on the cover, recalling a gold-tooled flying carpet. Published by a Boston drugstore, Clifford Pharmacy, it is an adventure story of travel to faraway places. The protagonists encounter perfume materials along the way—and quite fanciful stories about them, complete with woodcuts. One of the most imaginative is a poem about the tonka bean, the tale of a haughty and cruel princess who sends hundreds of men to their death in shark-infested waters as they compete for her hand in a swimming competition. Repentant, she drowns herself, and a tonka bean tree springs up in her place. Here are the final four stanzas of the dramatic seventeen-stanza poem.

From "The Legend of Beautiful Tonka"

Years having passed, the rolling tide
    From off that dreadful spot had dried;
When from the soil a shoot sprang forth, and grew
    Into a beauteous tree and bloomed,
    Its fruit full richly was perfumed;
Tree, bloom and fruit were very fair to view.

    And children played within its shade:
    One day a tiny little maid,
In joyous sport broke ope the nut-brown shell;
    When lo! before her enraptured eyes,
    To her great wonder and surprise,
Into her hand a tinier hand there fell.

    Go now, behold! this wondrous tree!
    And pluck its perfumed fruit, and see
That in each seed a maiden's hand there lies.
    'Tis for the swimmer bold, who died,
    And perished in that bloody tide,
A maiden's hand to gain; that tempting prize.

    'Tis thus we find the Tonka tree,
    Sprang from a maid beneath the sea;
Tonka, her name, means "fairest in the land."
    Redeemed, the maiden's pledge she gave,
    The while she sank beneath the wave,—
"I go to give my lovers, each, my hand."

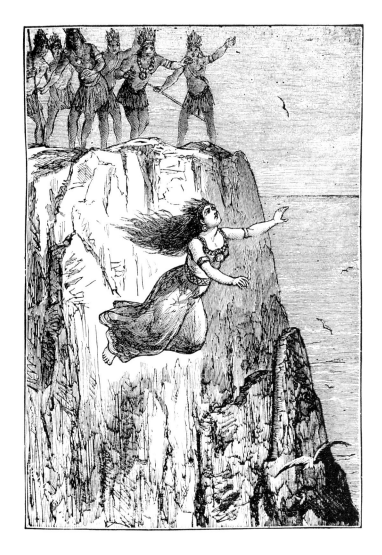

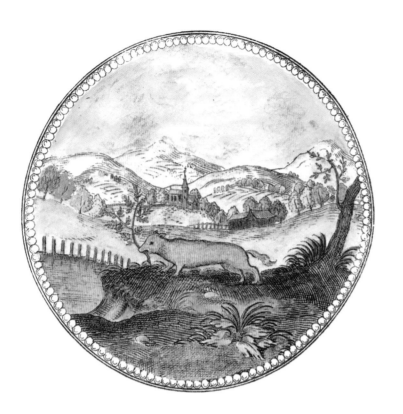

18
Hyraceum

The hyrax exhibit in the Aftel Archive.

At top are a hand-colored engraving of the klipdas, or southern African hyrax (see next spread) and an engraving of the daman, or Middle Eastern hyrax (France, 1760).

At bottom are pieces of hyraceum in a glass display case, an antique taxidermied hyrax from South Africa, and a hand-colored engraving of the southern African and Middle Eastern hyraxes (London, 1810).

The hyrax is a marvel of discovery and recycling. Rock hyraxes are native to Africa and the Middle East, living in colonies of ten to eighty individuals, all of whom have a habit of defecating and urinating in the same location. The gelatinous mixture of their excretions dries into a rock-like material—hyraceum—which is a sought-after ingredient in both traditional South African medicine and perfumery. It is rather miraculous that people somehow know to collect and use this substance.

The "stones" of hyraceum are brownish and brittle; when they are broken open, they release a dark oil with an intense, complex, fermented scent—sort of a cross between civet and castoreum. The mystery of how this was ever discovered and used in perfume opens up worlds of unknowable wonder inside your imagination: what could be beneath your feet, and in the trees, and everywhere in between?

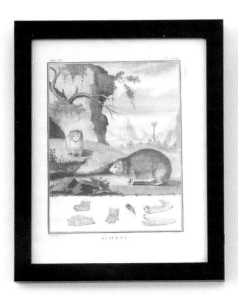

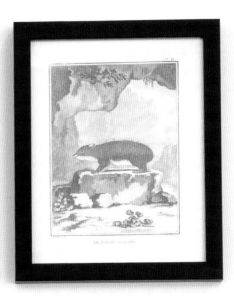

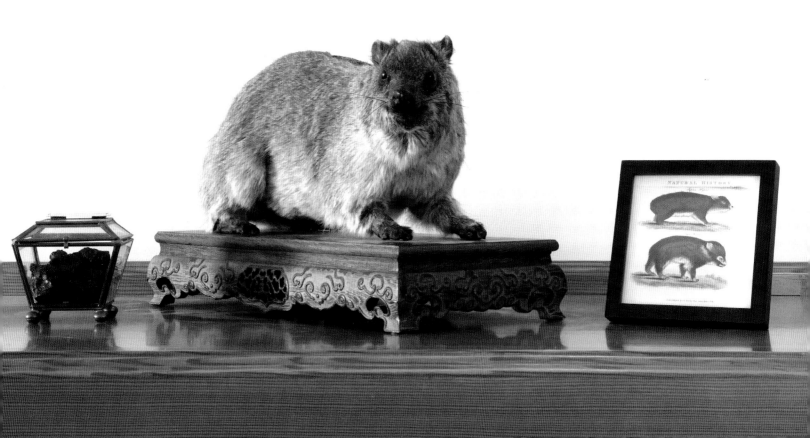

Funky and foul, hyraceum tempers sweetness in perfume, just as the bitter tempers sweetness in life.

Like the other animalic essences, hyraceum makes an excellent fixative in perfumery, and unlike some of the other animalic essences, it can be harvested without harming or intruding upon the species that produces it. The stones are still gathered by hand, as they have been since antiquity.

OPPOSITE
Hand-colored engraving of the klipdas, or southern African hyrax. Netherlands, 1783.

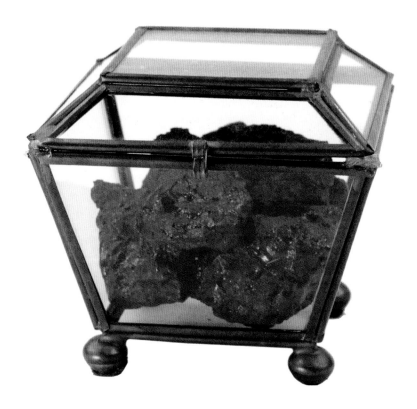

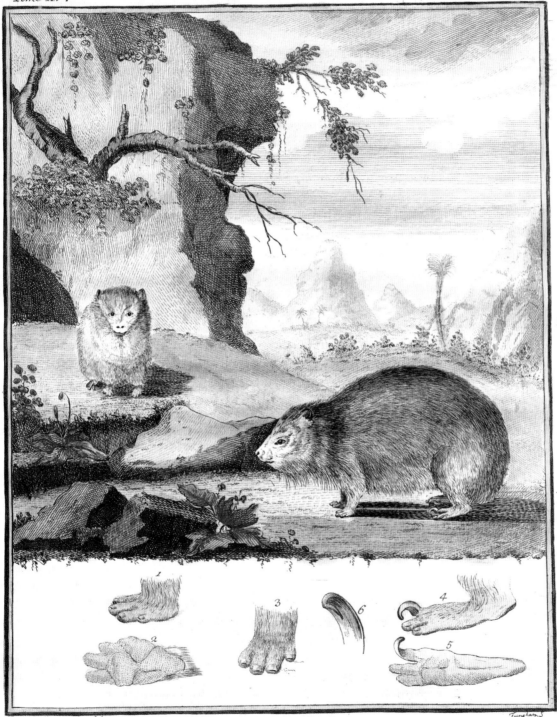

KLIPDAS.

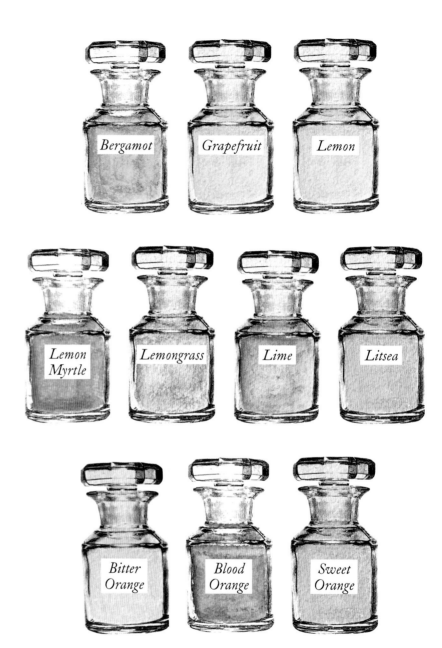

Bergamot

Grapefruit

Lemon

Lemon Myrtle

Lemongrass

Lime

Litsea

Bitter Orange

Blood Orange

Sweet Orange

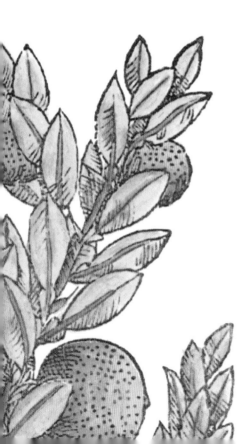

19
The
Citrus
Family

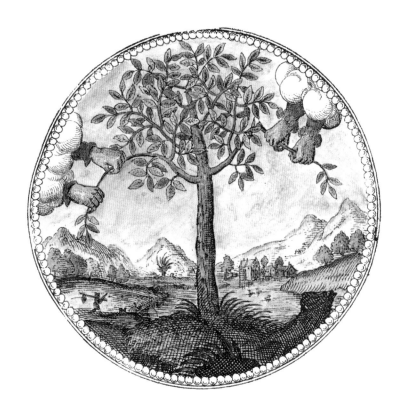

Citruses, as we know from everyday experience, are fragrant in all their parts—flowers, rind, and juice—but their essential oils are most heavily concentrated in the outer portion of the peel. If you press your fingernail into the peel of a citrus fruit, you will immediately come in contact with its essential oil. The best citrus oils are cold pressed, rather than distilled.

Citrus oils have much in common with each other: they are inexpensive, blend well with any other essence, and are top notes. They also have similar chemical makeups and are fairly close aromatically: they all provide freshness and brightness, and knit other essences together in a perfume. However, variations in certain trace components do create useful differences between them, and these can become major design considerations when designing a perfume. For example, oranges (except bitter orange) incline toward sweetness, lemon toward tartness, and grapefruit toward bitterness. Lemony aromas also appear prominently in non-citrus plants, broadening the possibilities of using a lemon scent.

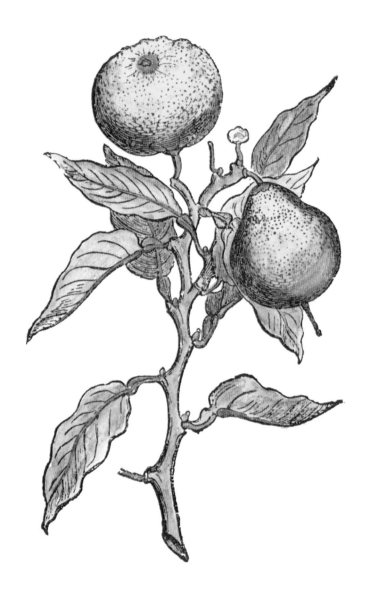

Bergamot

Citrus aurantium
subsp. *bergamia*
(or *Citrus bergamia*)

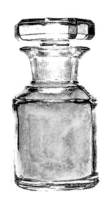

Bergamot is an inedible citrus fruit used exclusively for its delicate, bright, sweet, and slightly floral essential oil; it imparts pleasant, refreshing top notes with a floral back note. As the cornerstone of Chypre perfumes (a family of perfumes featuring the contrast of fresh bergamot and earthy oakmoss), bergamot has a long history in fragrance and is also the trademark flavor of Earl Grey tea. Bergamot is the only citrus that has more floral linalool than tart limonene. Welcome in any perfume, its special evanescent and ethereal quality distinguishes it from other citruses.

Available as an essential oil

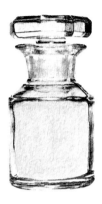

Grapefruit

Citrus ×paradisi

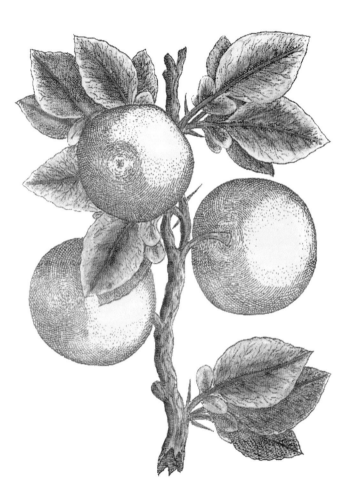

Bitter and acidic, grapefruit is eaten out of hand, often for breakfast. It is called grapefruit because the fruit grows in clusters, like grapes. The essential oil aroma has facets of pine, pear, and mango, and is the only citrus with coniferous notes. The most significant aroma molecule in grapefruit oil is nootkatone, which gives it a woody, cedarlike note. This is a great example of small aromatic facets making all the difference, because nootkatone constitutes only 0.2 percent of the aroma molecules in grapefruit essential oil. Without this smidge of nootkatone, a grapefruit would be more like an orange. Refreshing rather than dry, red grapefruit oil is sweeter than the white.

Available as an essential oil

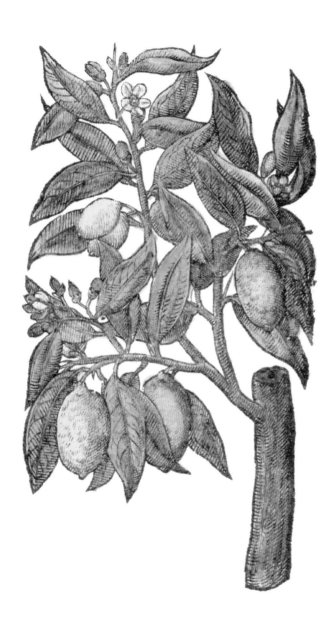

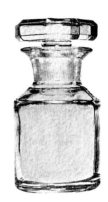

Lemon

Citrus limon

Lemon essential oil runs the risk of reminding people of toilet-bowl cleaner and furniture polish, because the scent of lemon has been so universal in those products. The uplifting smell of lemon is refreshingly sour and tart; it blends well with absolutely any other essence. The peel has the highest concentration of essential oils and delivers the most intense kick. Lemon is not especially dimensional in aroma, but it is almost universally welcome for its ability to bring lift, cut heaviness, and temper sweetness in a perfume.

Available as an essential oil

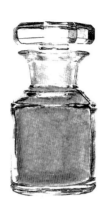

Lemon Myrtle

Backhousia citriodora

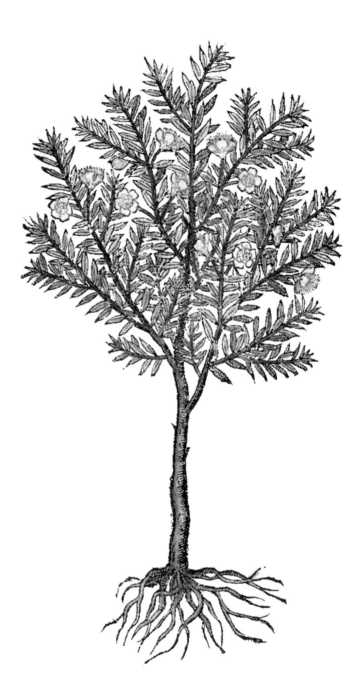

Distilled from the leaves of an evergreen tree, lemon myrtle has an intoxicating fresh, lemony smell—citrusy, but without the acidity. Prized by Australian Aborigines, it was used for cooking and, since it is strongly antibacterial, to treat wounds. From a genus named after Quaker missionary and botanist James Backhouse, it has eucalyptus herbal undertones, but the sharpness is softened by the presence of the aroma molecule linalool. In 1888, Schimmel & Co. isolated one of the first natural aroma molecules, citral, from lemon myrtle.

Available as an essential oil

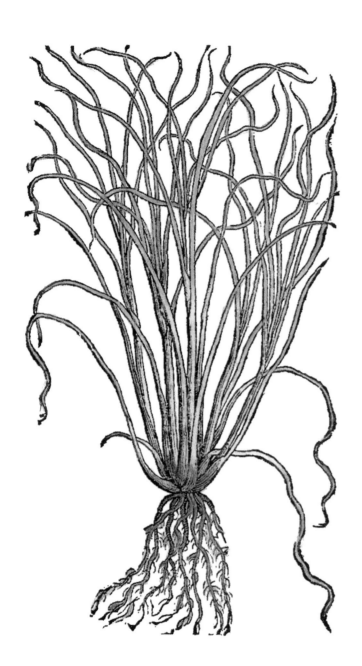

Lemon-grass

Cymbopogon citratus

The scientific name for lemongrass, *Cymbopogon*, is from the Greek words *kymbe*, "boat," and *pogon*, "beard," referring to the shape of its flowers, which resemble hairs springing from a boat-shaped sheath. It has been used for flavor for thousands of years in Asia, and in ancient Egypt the powdered root was used in perfumery. The aroma is a beautiful blend of fresh lemon, grassy, and herbaceous notes—like lemon verbena, but not as delicate.

Available as an essential oil

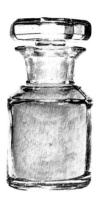

Lime

Citrus ×aurantifolia

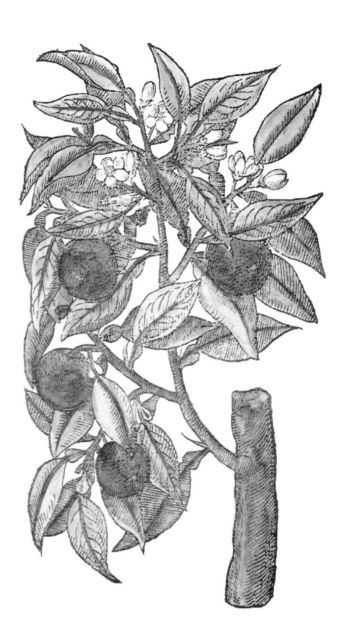

With its sweet, green, and spicy notes, lime is more rich, full-bodied, and aromatic than lemon. When combined with cinnamon oil, it is the foundation of all cola drinks. Lime oil gets along with any other essence in a blend and is perfect for extending green or fresh notes to the beginning of a perfume. Unlike lemon, lime is not associated with cleaning products, making it much more versatile in perfumery.

Available as an essential oil

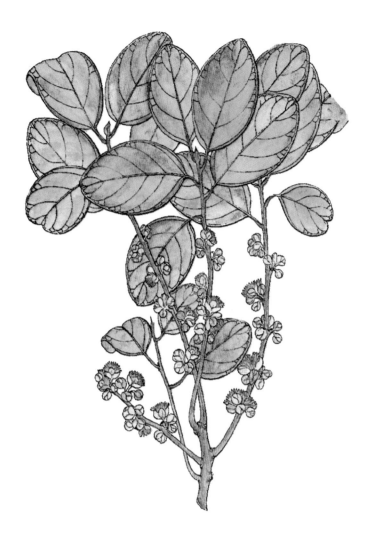

Litsea

Litsea cubeba

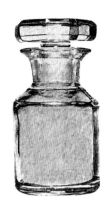

Litsea essential oil, distilled from the ripe fruits of the may chang plant, smells like lemon drop candy: sweet, fresh-but-tart lemon. In litsea, the bitterness of lemon is sweetened and tempered by floral geraniol molecules. The aroma has no bitter or grassy notes—just concentrated lemon with high odor intensity. Litsea is very useful in creating a perfume; since it is a middle note (unlike most citruses, which are top notes), it allows you to add a citrus facet to floral middle notes.

Available as an essential oil

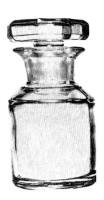

Bitter Orange

Citrus ×aurantium

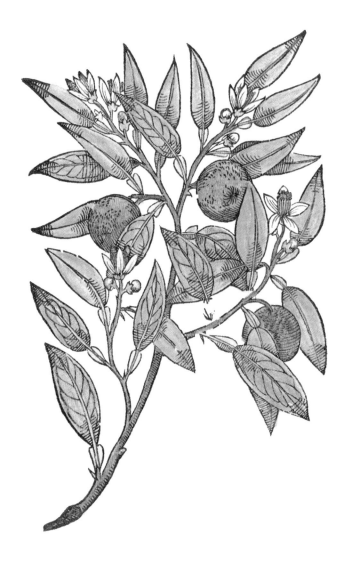

Bitter orange oil is acidic, fresh yet bitter, and slightly floral. Sometimes called sour orange, it is dry but with the characteristic brightness of orange. Petitgrain oil is distilled from the leaves and twigs of the same tree, and its aroma is woodier and drier than the one expressed from the peel.

Limonene is the dominant aroma molecule in all orange essential oils, but sweet orange has facets of lemon (citral) and floral (linalool), whereas bitter orange has a larger floral (linalool) facet, and blood orange has berry facets. By choosing among the different orange aromas, you can slant your fragrance toward sweet and complex (sweet orange), floral and dry (bitter orange), or a rich berry (blood orange).

Available as an essential oil

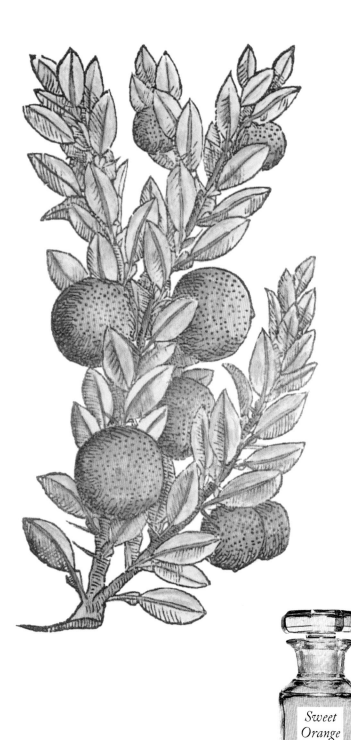

Blood and Sweet Orange

Citrus ×sinensis

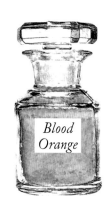

Blood Orange

Sweet orange is one of the most popular smells and tastes in the world. The fruit, eaten fresh out of hand, is sweet—as opposed to lemon, which is used for flavoring but too sour to be eaten. Since the thirteenth century, sweet orange has been the most important and widely cultivated of all the citrus flavors. Its aroma is heavy, rich, sweet yet fresh, bright, and powerful.

Blood orange has ruby-streaked flesh and berry notes, and smells like a mix between sweet oranges and raspberries. Its aroma is stronger and more pronounced than sweet or bitter orange.

Available as essential oils

Sweet Orange

20
Floral
Reverie

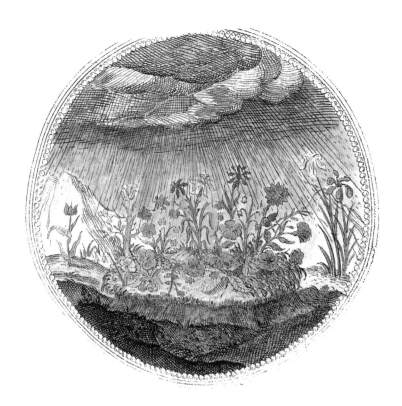

Postcards are tentative travelers, incomplete until someone receives them. Printed photographs enabled a visitor to share with a special someone far away images of the collecting and processing of flowers for use in perfume—violets, cassia, narcissus, tuberose, rose, orange flower, and jasmine—at Grasse, the famous perfume center in southern France. To a modern-day observer, though, these postcards convey not only information about another era, but its sensibilities. They reveal the devotion to a craft that was then really based on— inspired by—natural essences.

These images are not static: the hand-tinted photographs elevate documentation into the lyrical domain of painting. Inducing an imaginative reverie, these magical images speak of a time when the gathering and processing of aromatic materials was beautiful, poetic, and artisanal. Working by hand created a deep connection to the land and plants and seasons. Witnessing these scenes brings alive the centuries-old process of using plants to create perfume.

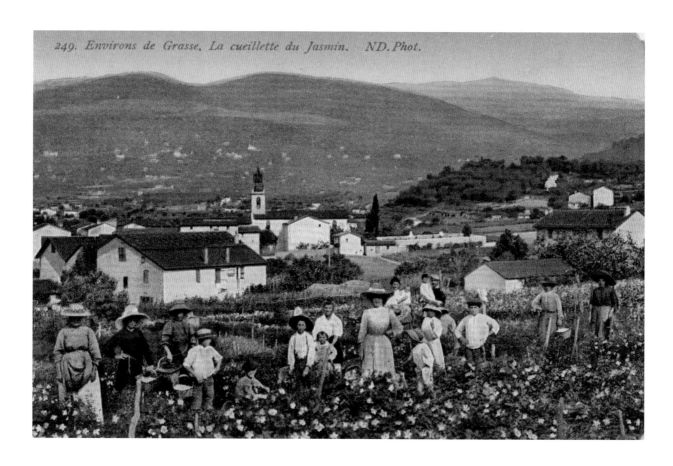

249. *Environs de Grasse. La cueillette du Jasmin.* ND. Phot.

Scents are one of the most subtle and delicate charms of life. They come to us in the solemn silence of nature. They awaken sensibility, stir the mind, stimulate the imagination, and revive memory. Their importance to body and soul has been emphasized by every civilization and every religion in every part of the world. They float between reality and transcendence, between matter and spirit.

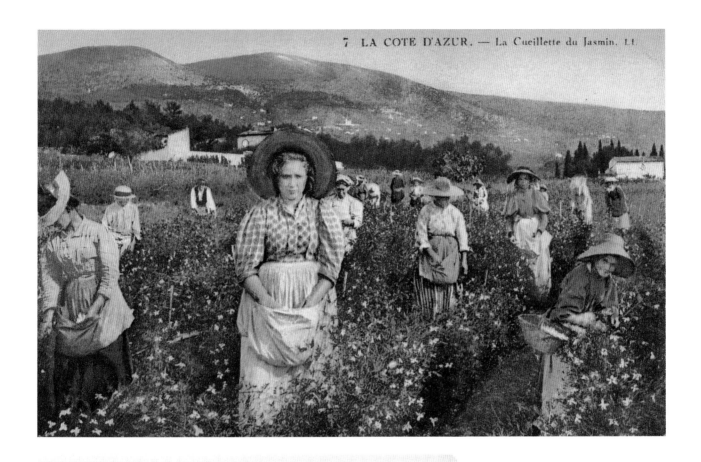

7   LA COTE D'AZUR. — La Cueillette du Jasmin. Lt.

The word "essence," which is in all probability derived from the Latin word esse, meaning "to be," takes us far back in the history of man's thought and endeavours to those days when science and superstition were closely intertwined. The old alchemists commonly believed that every substance had a soul: to obtain the soul of a substance was to obtain that substance in its full potency.

—H. Stanley Redgrove, *Spices and Condiments*, 1933

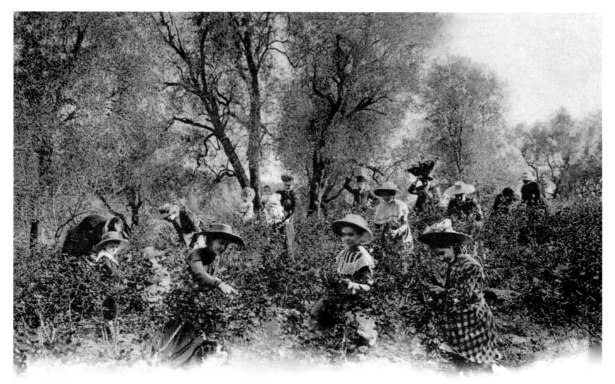

COTE D'AZUR — Cueillette des roses

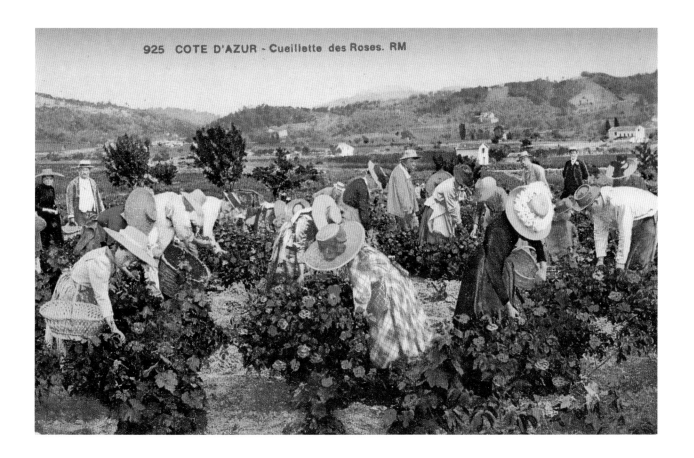

925 COTE D'AZUR - Cueillette des Roses. RM

These abundant flowers are collected and turned into con-centrated essences for use in perfume. Essences contain the plant's entire life history. All of the materials that created it live on in the bottle: the soil where it grew, the water it drank, the breezes that blew on it—each leave their traces in its unique scent. Each plant essence contains dozens or even hundreds of aroma molecules, blended over time to create a unique aromatic signature. Nature is the original perfumer!

ABOVE AND OPPOSITE
Collecting roses

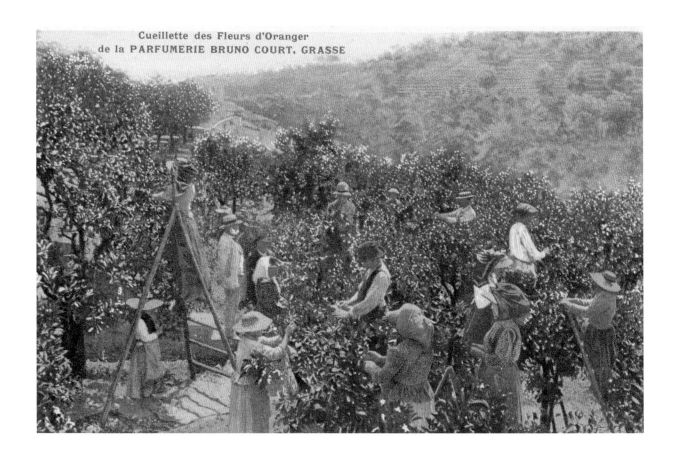

Cueillette des Fleurs d'Oranger
de la PARFUMERIE BRUNO COURT, GRASSE

ABOVE AND OPPOSITE
Collecting orange blossoms

Floral essences are alive, and they stay alive forever, deepening and evolving; they come to us from a kind of afterlife, like something divine. Even the most fleeting and transitory aspects of the plant's existence are miraculously captured in them. They are, in a sense, life eternal, reincarnate, and they permeate (literally) every spiritual tradition.

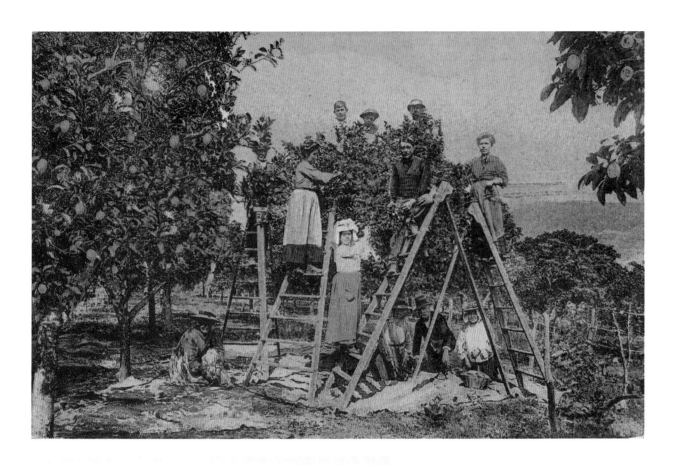

Then were not summer's distillation left,
A liquid prisoner pent in walls of glass,
Beauty's effect with beauty were bereft,
Nor it, nor no remembrance what it was:
But flowers distilled, though they with winter meet,
Leese but their show; their substance still lives sweet.
　　—Shakespeare, Sonnet V

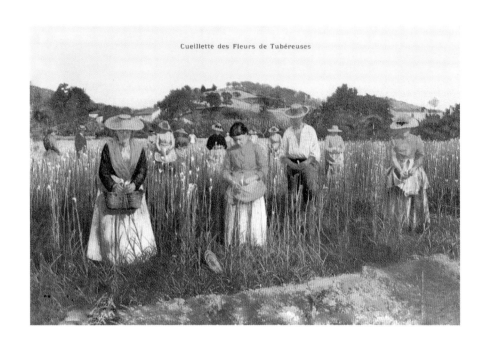

Cueillette des Fleurs de Tubéreuses

THIS PAGE
Collecting tuberose

OPPOSITE
Collecting violets

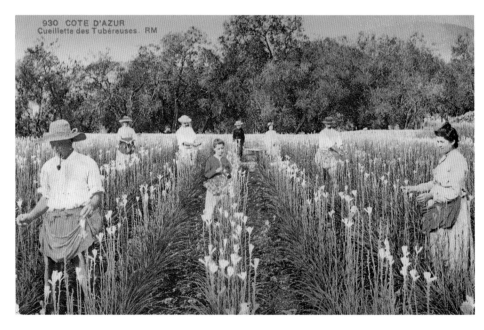

930 COTE D'AZUR
Cueillette des Tubéreuses. RM

The plant's natural life cycle is limited, but it lives on in its essences. They capture the ongoing blooming of the rose, the flow of sap in the tree, the sprouting of the seed in the ground. In the scent bottle, the bliss of the garden is eternal: no dusk will arrive, no rain will fall.

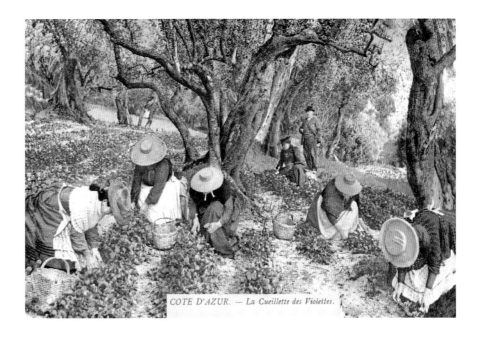

COTE D'AZUR. — *La Cueillette des Violettes.*

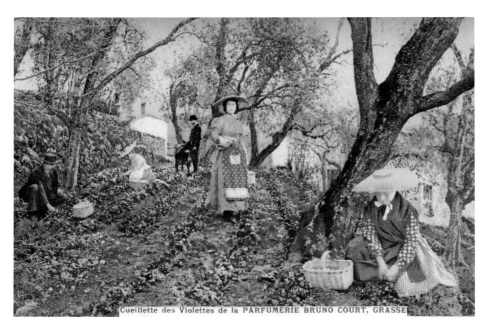

Cueillette des Violettes de la PARFUMERIE BRUNO COURT, GRASSE

Floral Abundance

OPPOSITE TOP
Piles of roses

OPPOSITE BOTTOM
Hard at work on geranium

When viewing these representations of things that really happened, we also experience them as a dream—a daydream in which we ourselves journey in our imagination: we are in the presence of the people, the landscapes, the machines, the piles of petals. A scene on which we meditate is at once outside of us and the image of our interiority; it draws us deep into our imagination.

These postcards of piles of flowers used to create essences for perfume are an astounding and overwhelming image of abundance. To let yourself enter any of these photographs is to swim in a sea of odoriferous molecules, beauteous beyond belief and gorgeous in their coloration and texture. It is the essence of perfume. These postcards give us a sense of the vast amount of material needed and used—the abundance that was there in the harvesting. Imagine what the air in the room smelled like, as workers waded through the mounds of flowers on the floor.

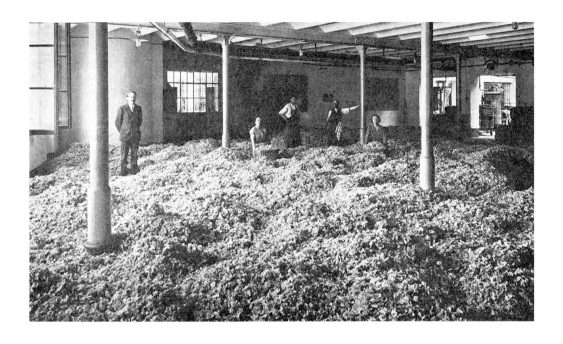

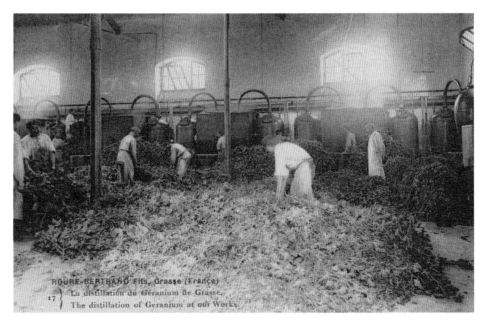

ROURE-BERTRAND Fils, Grasse (France)
La distillation du Géranium de Grasse.
17 The distillation of Geranium at our Works.

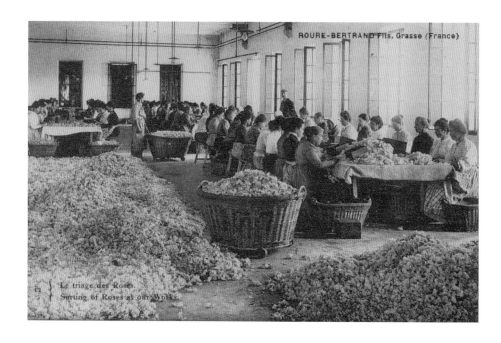

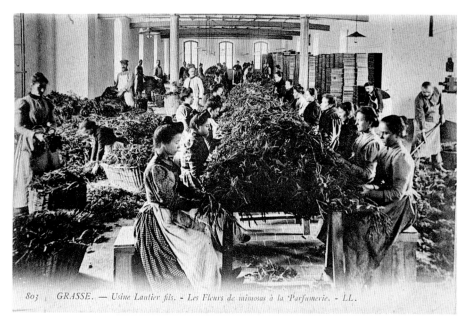

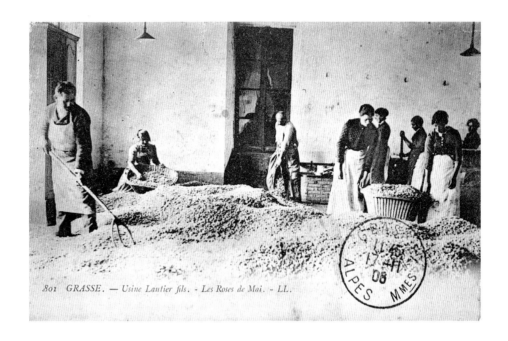

801 GRASSE. — Usine Lautier fils. - Les Roses de Mai. - LL.

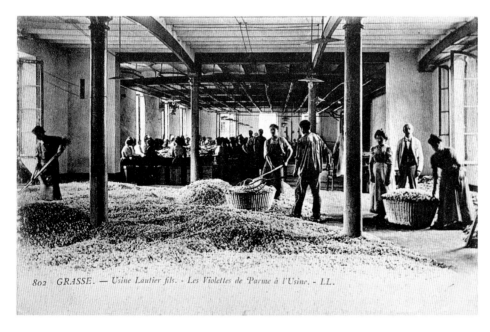

802 GRASSE. — Usine Lautier fils. - Les Violettes de Parme à l'Usine. - LL.

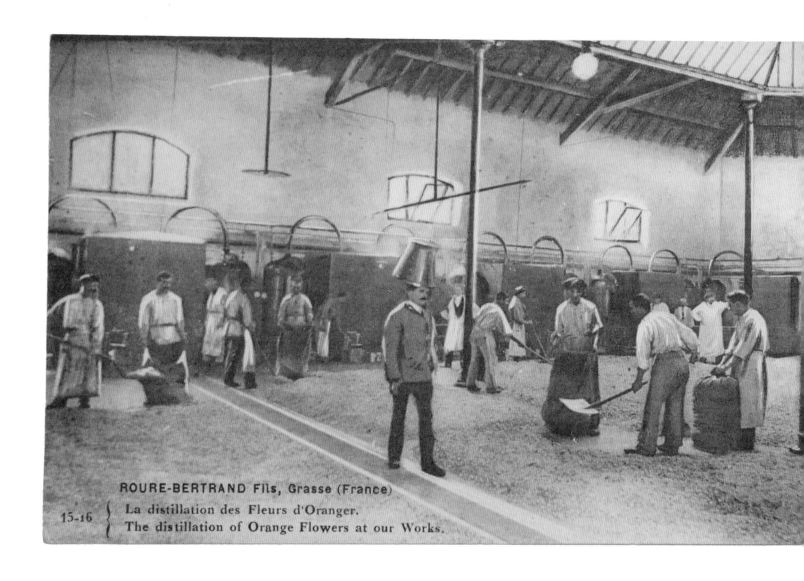

ROURE-BERTRAND Fils, Grasse (France)

15-16 { La distillation des Fleurs d'Oranger.
The distillation of Orange Flowers at our Works.

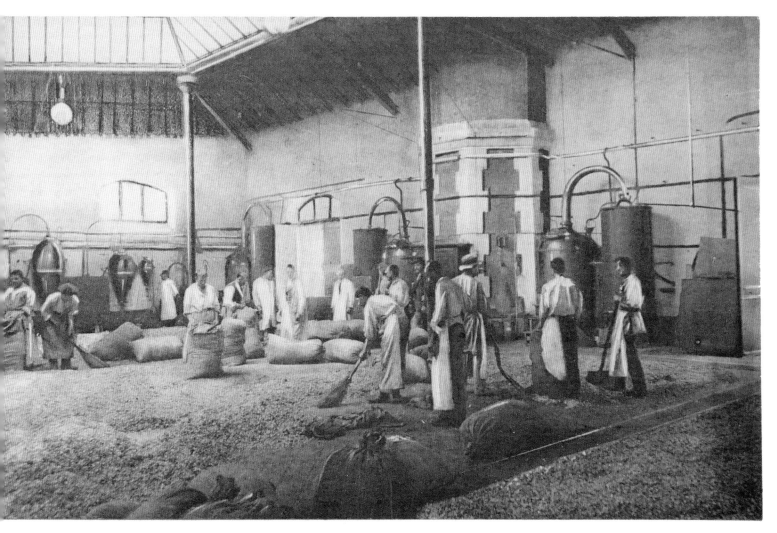

Wall-to-wall orange blossom panorama

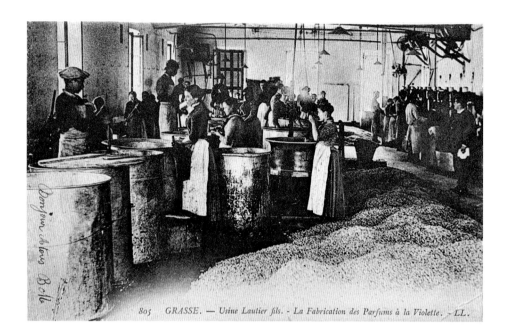

805 GRASSE. — Usine Lautier fils. - La Fabrication des Parfums à la Violette. - LL.

Wading in violets

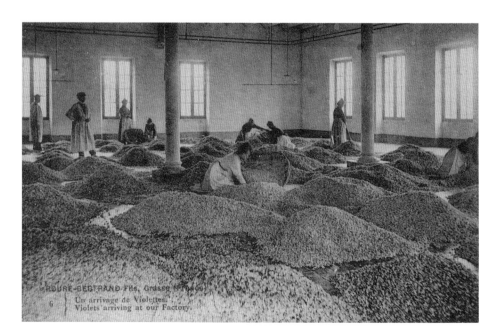

ROURE-BERTRAND Fils, Grasse
Un arrivage de Violettes.
Violets arriving at our Factory.

Swimming in violets

21
Castoreum

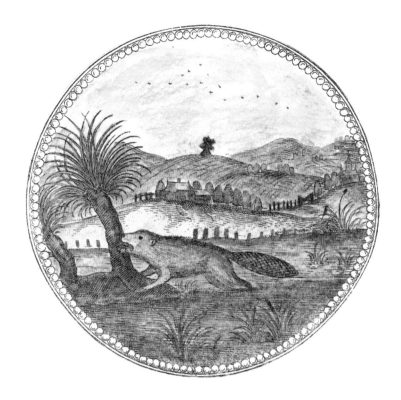

In perfumery, castoreum has been used as the key scent in classic leather-themed perfumes—evocative of fine leather goods. The deep, smoky aroma, considered an aphrodisiac, contributes an erotic, spicy, ambery note to perfumes, as well as providing fixation. Castoreum is also used to fortify bourbon whiskey and to add a leathery raspberry taste to food.

Castoreum is a thick paste found in the castor sacs of the beaver, which are present in both males and females between the pelvis and the base of the tail. The beavers themselves, notoriously territorial and aggressive toward intruders, use it to scent-mark, constructing scent mounds made of mud, debris, and castoreum along the border of their territory.

Nowadays, regions with large native beaver populations typically have an open trapping season to limit the damage caused by overpopulation of the species. The castor sacs are either smoked or dried in the sun, and as they age, they look like very large, dried figs; meanwhile, the aroma of the castoreum mellows into a smell of sweet, clean leather.

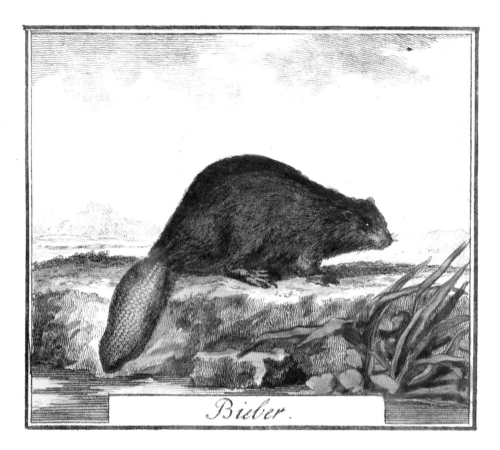

Bieber.

OPPOSITE

The castoreum exhibit in the museum: a papier-mâché beaver by Erin Cramer, 2016; a hundred-year-old Dodge and Olcott castoreum bottle; castor sacs containing castoreum

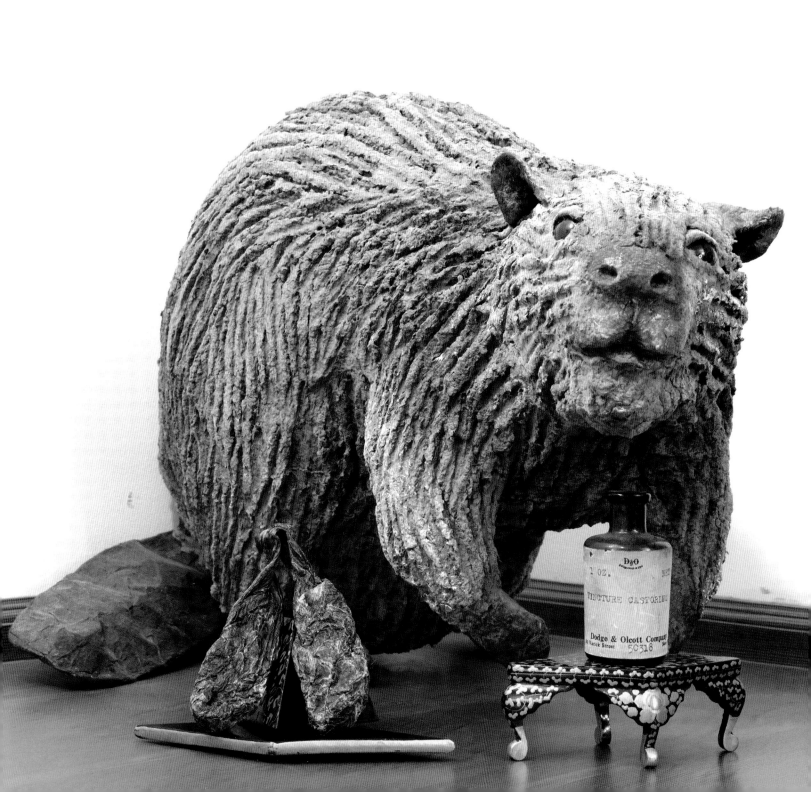

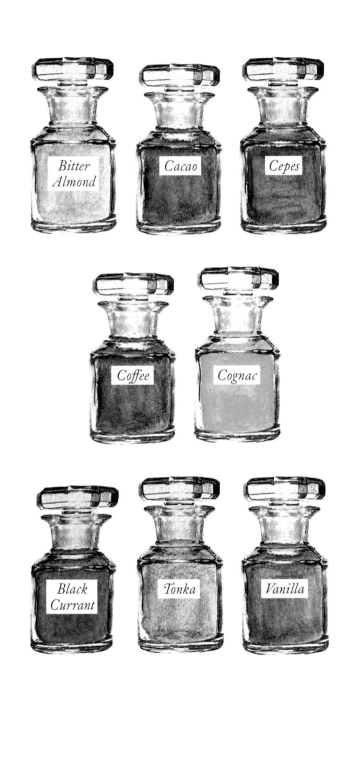

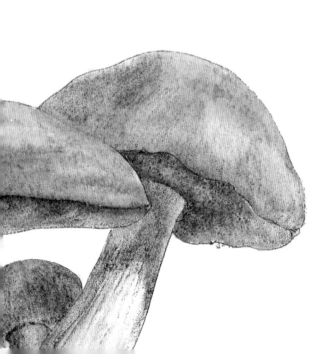

22
The Gourmand Family

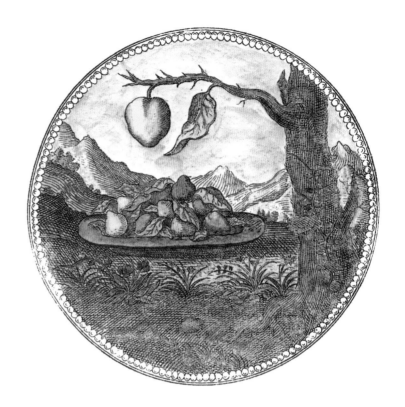

Many aromas that we think of as primarily connected to something edible find their way into perfume. Cake, cookies, coffee, mushrooms, caramel, candy, and chocolate are as enjoyable to smell as they are to eat. The rich and delicious essences in this family remind us of food and drink, and their complex aromas create strange magic when combined with florals, fruits, and spices. When you smell these essences, you need to free them from their strictly culinary identity and reacquaint yourself with the complexity and beauty of their individual aromas.

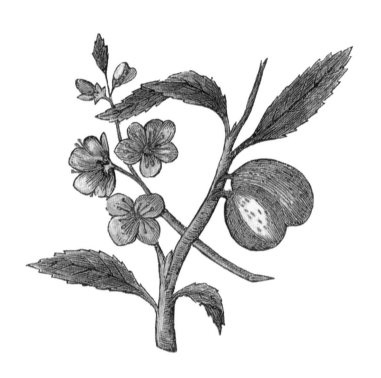

Bitter Almond

Prunus amygdalus

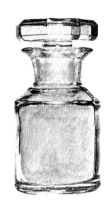

Bitter almond's sweet cherry aroma, both floral and fruity, is known for its ability to help mimic most floral scents. Almost every antique perfume book relies on bitter almond essential oil to re-create the scents of single flowers that cannot be harvested from nature. The aroma molecule benzaldehyde makes up 97 percent of the essential oil, which has a very high odor intensity and should be used sparingly in any fragrance. Bitter almond extract, which lends its marzipan flavor to cookies and cakes, is made from the essential oil tinctured in alcohol.

Available as an essential oil

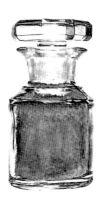

Cacao

Theobroma cacao

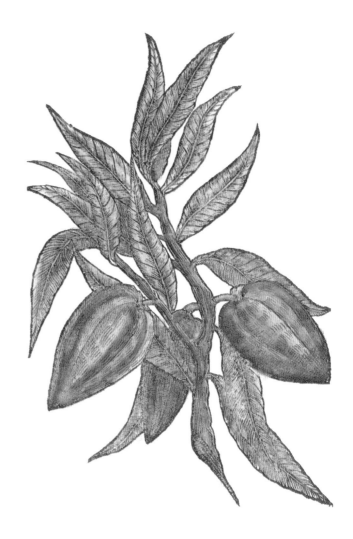

Chocolate is made from the processed seeds of the fruit pod of the cacao tree. The ripe pods are spectacular: seven to twelve inches long, reddish brown to purple, with a pale pink to soft whitish pulp inside that contains the seeds. The aroma is dark, earthy, and rich, like wild mushrooms; it can be used to modify almost any floral essence, making it dirtier and sexier without any real reference to the common sweet dessert aspect of chocolate.

Available as an absolute

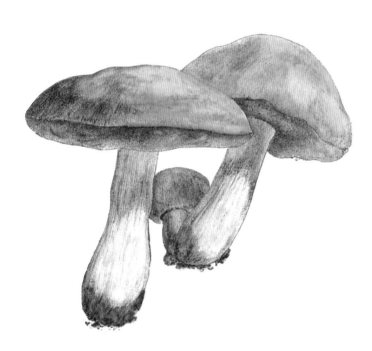

Cepes

Boletus edulis

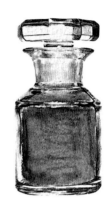

Cepes, or porcini mushrooms, grow symbiotically with tree roots and have the intense, earthy, fungal aroma characteristic of wild mushrooms. Used sparingly, cepes absolute helps ground floral notes with earthy and dirty facets. The aroma is complex and multifaceted, with aspects of moss and earth, specifically the dirt that clings to roots. Surprisingly, this rich, dark aroma is also reminiscent of dark chocolate. Cepes can be used to mimic animal essences.

Available as an absolute

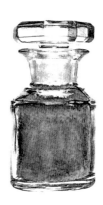

Coffee

Coffee arabica and
robusta (or *canephora*)

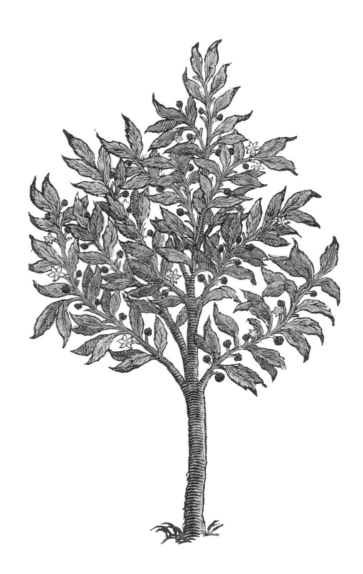

Coffee began in ancient times as a food. It was introduced as a beverage in the thirteenth century in Turkey, and the first coffeehouse in Italy was opened in 1645. The popularity of the beverage was immediate and enormous, quickly spreading around the world.

The coffee scent only develops as the beans age and are roasted. Coffee essence's earthy and dark aroma is useful to counter excessive sweetness in a perfume. When you pry the aroma of coffee free from its identity as a popular beverage, you will discover a dark, dank, rich aroma reminiscent of the earth beneath our feet.

Available as a CO_2 and an essential oil. The CO_2 has a cleaner aroma, roasted but not cooked.

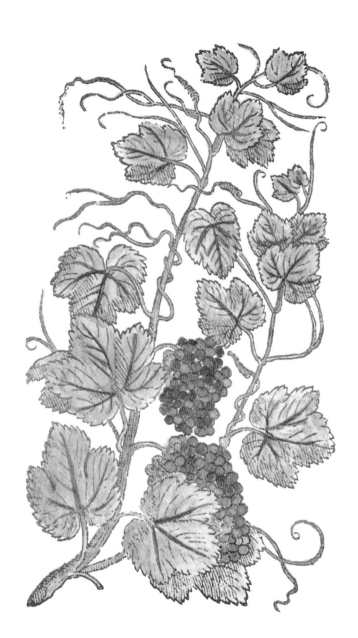

Cognac

Vitis vinifera

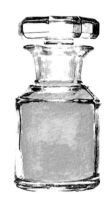

Cognac essential oil is produced by steam distilling the lees left from the fermentation of grape brandy—a perfect example of upcycling leftovers. The oil is a significant aromatic component of cognac itself; it has great diffusive power and provides lift to a perfume composition. Cognac provides unique blending possibilities: it is the only intensely fruity (green apple-y) note in a natural perfumer's palette. With facets of vanilla (vanillin), plummy rose (damascenone), and whiskey (guaiacol), the aroma is layered and complex, like fine wine.

Available as green cognac essential oil (sweeter) and white cognac essential oil (drier)

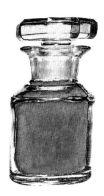

Black Currant

Ribes nigrum

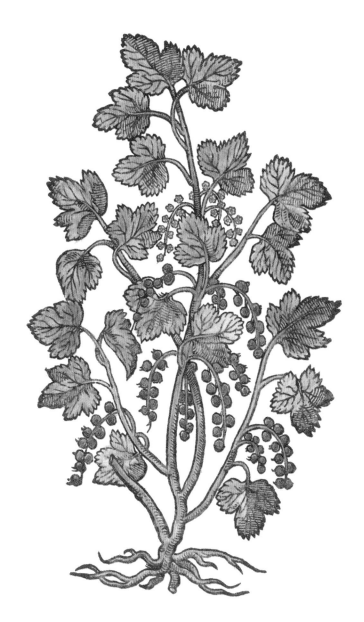

The young leaves and berries of black currant, and most especially the fresh flower buds, contain the intensely fragrant odoriferous glands. Black currant is a very complex, powerful, and somewhat strange aroma: besides being jammy and fruity, it has undertones of sulphur and musk—and cat pee! This very tangy catty note is due to the presence of thiols, which are also found in cat urine.

Available as an absolute

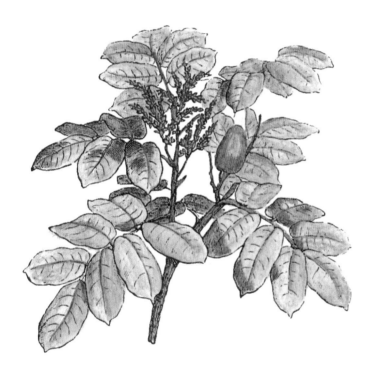

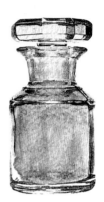

Tonka

Dipteryx odorata

The caramel, sweet powdery smell of tonka comes from its predominant aroma molecule, coumarin. With its smell of new-mown hay, coumarin was the first aroma molecule to be synthesized, in 1868, and ushered in the world of synthetic perfumery. Once people understood that they could make natural aromas synthetically for much less money, the world of perfume changed forever! Tonka is the utimate powdery vanilla note, making a perfume softer and warmer.

Available as an absolute

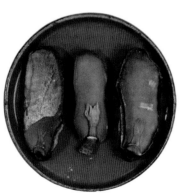

Tonka bean "hands" inside some samples in the museum

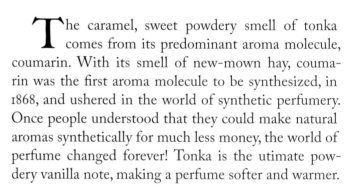

We noticed something very curious in connection with these beans, on equally dividing one perpendicularly; at the lower part of the bean, that part where it was attached to the branch, is a tiny hand, showing the fingers perfectly, and a small part of the arm, seemingly encircled by a bracelet

—F. S. Clifford, *Romance of Perfume Lands*, 1881

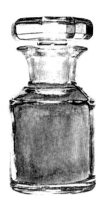

Vanilla

Vanilla planifolia

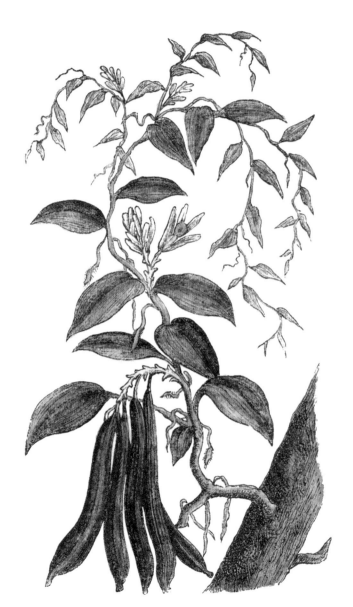

Vanilla seed pods have no fragrance when they are gathered, but develop their characteristic odor during the curing process. By degrees the color darkens, the flesh softens, and the true odor of vanilla begins to develop as the natural fermentation gradually progresses up the pod, which takes about a month. Vanilla's addictive aroma is smooth, sweet, and balsamic, with cherry undertones. Although the naturally occurring molecule vanillin is the most important component of vanilla beans, the gorgeous aroma and taste of vanilla, like those of so many essences, are composed of nature's own mixture of major and minor constituents.

In 1874, synthetic vanillin was the second aroma molecule to be synthesized, which helped usher in the world of cheap synthetic essences for creating sweetness in flavor and perfume. However, real vanilla has nothing in common with the insipid synthetic vanilla that is so pervasive in perfumes and body products. Real vanilla is balsamic, woody, raisiny, rich, complex, and beloved.

Available as an absolute and a CO_2 extract

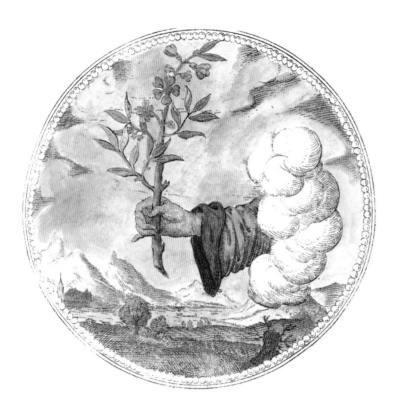

23
Maker's Knowledge

Pastilles
1 ʒ Benzoin 4 ʒ Styrax 4 ʒ Cloves 12 Charcoal
1 ʒ Gum Dragon 1 ʒ Oil Lavender

Pastilles Fine

4 ʒ Benzoin 4 ʒ Styrax 1 Drm Rhodium
1 ʒ Balsam of Peru 6 oʒ Charcoal
½ ʒ Es of Ambergris 12 ʒ Gum dragon
½ Pint orange flower water 1 drm Neroli

A handwritten recipe book documents a maker's knowledge and experience of materials in their own hand—the same hand that did the making. The intimacy of their ink, pen, or even manual typewriter is personal yet universal. The recipes in these books—for perfumes, dyes, medicine, remedies—all share an intimate connection and reverence for the natural botanical materials.

Handwritten American formula book of perfumes and household items, 1838

Ghostly apparitions of script, each letter carefully rendered

Vanilla powder recipe from the 1838 formula book

Whoever wrote this knew what she was doing! This recipe is complicated and sophisticated, and it was probably intended for a potpourri: orris powder—a soft violet aroma—is perfect for smoothing the vanilla, and it is clever to broaden it by adding tonka, a sweet, caramelly variation on vanilla. And benzoin adds another vanilla facet, showing a further acumen and familiarity with the ingredients.

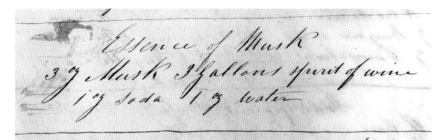

Essence of Musk
3 ℥ Musk 2 Gallons spirit of wine
1 ℥ Soda 1 ℥ Water

Ambergris Essence
1 Pt spirit 1 drm Neroli 1 ℥ Musk ½ ℥ Amber
4 ℥ Orris 4 ℥ Jonquil 2 ℥ Jasmin 2 ℥ Tuberose

Ess of Musk ought to stand one year

Ambergris and musk essences
in the 1838 formula book

I want to meet this woman! She has an unbelievable supply of materials in her house that she seems to know how to work with. How did she procure the ambergris *and* musk (*and* civet) in her home, aging for years?

Cologne Mixture
2 Gallon Alkohol
5 oz Bergamotte
5 " Lemon
1 oz Lavender Flour
1 " Petit Grain
½ oz Neroli
2½ oz Benjoin Tincture

Perfume for Common Cost
1½ oz. Ess. Bergamotte
3½ " Lavender Flour
3½ " Rosemary
4 oz Spermint
8 " Cloves.

Woodworths fine Cologne
5 Gallon Alkohol
2 oz Neroli
2 " Rosemary
4 " Bergamotte
4 " Lemon
4 " Orange
½ Gallon Aqua
4. 20.

Fine Cologne for Pitch
15 Gallon Alkohol
8 oz Lavender Flour
8 oz Bergamotte
8 " Lemon
3 " Citronelle
2 " Rosemary
4 " Cassie
2 oz Cloves
5 Gallon Aqua

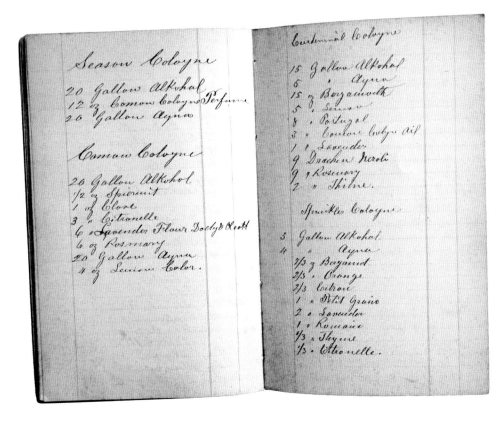

German Cologne No 1

9 Gallon Alkohol
5½ oz Neroli
3 " Rosemary
8 " Orange
6 " Lemon
8 " Bergamotte
1 Gallon Ayua
        4.80.

German Cologne No 2.

9 Gallon Alkohol
3 oz Petit Grain
6 " Bergamotte
3 oz Rosemary
6 " Orange
6 " Lemon
4 oz Neroli
1 Gallon Ayua
        3. 30.

Sprinkling Cologne

24 Gallon Alkohol
16 oz Comon Cologne Perfume
1 oz Thine
1 " Citeonelle
16 Gallon Ayua
2 oz Yellow Color.
        1.54

Florida Water.

15 Gallon Alkohol   37
12 oz Bergauotte   3   38
8 " Orange   1   25
4 " Lemon   1   00
1 " Cloves   21
4 " Civette   24
1 " Petit grain   80
2 " Lavender Flour   25
1/2 " Peppermint   13
1 Gallon Orris   3   00
1 " Ambette   3   70
7 " Ayua
2 oz Yellow color   5
        2. 20

Season Cologne

20 Gallon Alkohol
12 oz Comon Cologne Perfume
20 Gallon Ayua

Comon Cologne

20 Gallon Alkohol
1/2 oz Spiermint
1 oz Clove
3 " Citeonelle
6 " Lavender Flour Dodey & Scott
6 oz Rosmary
20 Gallon Ayua
4 oz Lemon Color.

Centennial Cologne

15 Gallon Alkohol
5 " Ayua
15 oz Bergauotte
5 " Lemon
8 " Portugal
3 " Centur Cologne Oil
1 " Lavender
9 Drachm Neroli
9 " Rosmary
2 " Thine.

Sprinkle Cologne

5 Gallon Alkohol
4 " Ayua
2/3 oz Bergamot
2/3 " Orange
2/3 Citron
1 " Petit Grain
2 " Lavender
1 " Romain
1/3 " Thyme
1/3 " Citeonelle.

Recipe notebook, 1876

This perfumer is very thorough if not compulsive in these explorations in her notebook, trying to understand how to make colognes. Working with citruses, subtly shading them with herbs, making different variations—all go to show that these recipes were worked out by hand with a real passion.

Narcissus - very pleasant. Another species, Narcissus Jonquilla found on market as extract etc, of Jonquil are artificial compounds.

Nutmeg - used in perfumery, rarely pure, mostly in combination with other strong odors.

Olibanum - used for incense for religious purposes, & fumigating. Pleasant though faint odor.

Orange Flowers - very fragrant essential oil. (Leaves used - contain a peculiar ... used in perfumery.

Orange Peel - in perfumery & liqueurs.

Orris Root - used for sachets & fixing other odors.

Palm Oil - cheap perfumes.

Patchouly - East Indian & Chinese Goods, such as shawls, etc owe their peculiar odor to patchouly herb.

Peru Balsam - odor agreeable & balsamic.

Pink - genuine odor of Pinks, sold under this name usually artificial mixtures of other odors.

Plumeria - sometimes called Frangipanni, is made of combination of different odors.

Reseda (mignonette) refreshing. True odor of Reseda is very expensive for this reason nearly all perfume sold under that name are aromatic substances.

Rhodium - (Bois de rose) odor resembles that of rose.

Rose - The wild rose, sweet brier, French eglantine, possesses a delicate but very fugitive odor, & perfume sold as wild rose, is usually prepared from other substances with the addition of oil of rose. The same applies to the odor called "white rose", "tea rose" "moss rose" etc.

Rosemary - refreshing odor, frequently added in small amounts to fine perfumes.

Rue - strong odor. Used occasionally in perfumes.

Sage - suitable for sachets, tooth powders etc.

Santal-Wood - very fragrant, also called sandal-wood. White or yellow santal wood resembles oil of rose. (Reddish-brown santal-wood used only for coloring perfumes.)

Sassafras - for soaps, flavorings.

Star - Anise - liqueurs, & perfumery.

Storax - has the peculiar property of binding different, very delicate odors, to render them less fugitive. (Belongs among the balsams - & obtained from bark

INSTRUCTIONS FOR MIXING PERFUMES.

Perfumers mix their ingredients by several methods. When experimenting with an original bouquet, they generally build directly from the absolute oils, animal fixatives and synthetics adding alcohol to small batches before aging. Thus they can test as they go, without great expenditure of time. Other perfumers add to the alcohol only the animal fixatives and the absolute oils, and then, after aging, slowly and carefully experiment with the addition of synthetics, and later with natural oils; thus they will enlarge the harmony until a new bouquet appears. Still other perfumers begin with the alcohol and synthetics, introducing the floral and animal odors last. These perfumers lean heavily on the synthetics; they claim that the highest perfume artistry is that which only falls back on (expensive) floral absolutes when the possibilities of the synthetics have been exhausted. They rely on the natural essence and animal fixative only to finish the perfume with a soft, resonant tone and attenuating echo. Let your nose be your guide to your method. The proper combination of odors requires a natural gift that cannot be instilled by any amount of instruction. But you will never know whether you have an undetected genius for perfumery until you test it.

Perfumer's notebook, handwritten and typed, Erie, Pennsylvania, 1937

The diary of this anonymous self-taught perfumer, working with naturals and synthetics, follows the workings of his mind as he develops his craft, revealing great research and a deep knowledge of materials. This activity is timeless—the process he was carrying out then is the same in spirit as what I do now, almost a hundred years later, in my studio.

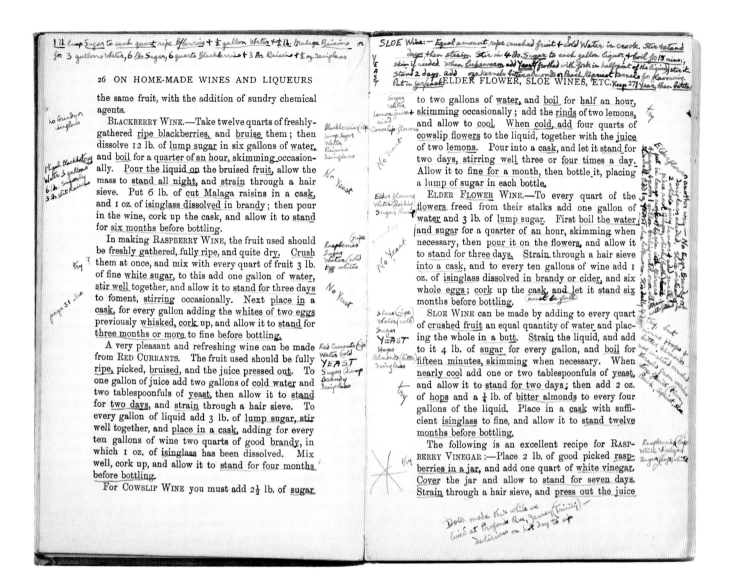

C. J. S. Thompson,
Housewife's Handy-Book, *1896*

The owner's copious notes and handwritten annotations of what worked (and what didn't) make this book her own. The tiny, meticulous handwriting, the careful study of the recipes, the window into the process as they become her own are enchanting.

2 double or jacketed pans with lids, 2 shallow enamelled pans, 4 small enamelled pans, 1 pestle and mortar, No. 6 Wedgewood; 4 white earthenware bowls of various sizes, 1 set of fluid measures (half-

She notes her desire for a pestle and mortar from the list of recommended equipment.

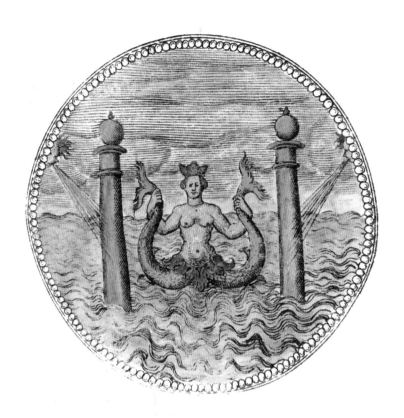

24
Onycha

"One can therefore compare this unguis [onycha] with a basse in Musick which when heard alone has no comliness, but when mixed with other voices, makes for a sweet accord, maintains the same."
—Rumphius, *The Ambonese Curiosity Cabinet*, 1705

O nycha, an aromatic used in incense since ancient times, is derived from the flap that closes the outer shell of an edible marine mollusk. Displayed in a bowl in the museum, these shells beckon to be handled, creating a clatter of castanets. Like all other animal essences, onycha brings out the animalic aspects and increases the longevity of a perfume.

Onycha smells leathery and animalic, recalling the scent of the sea and brine. The traditional Indian essence *choya nakh* is made from onycha shells that have been broken into chunks and roasted; the aroma smells like a campfire on the beach.

OPPOSITE
The onycha exhibit in the Aftel Archive. On the wall are two antique prints of onycha, reproduced on the next spread. On the shelf, left to right, are a basket of medium onycha shells, a large onycha shell, and a hand-colored woodcut of Onycha (German, 1600).

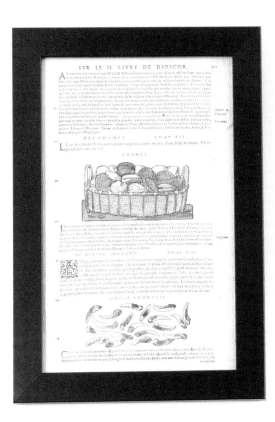

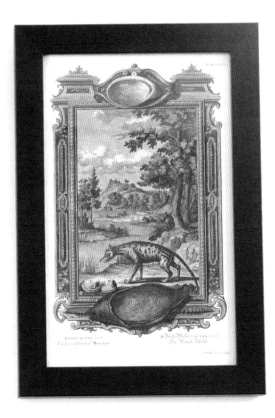

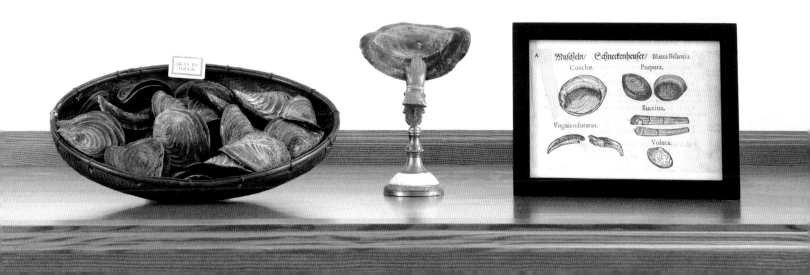

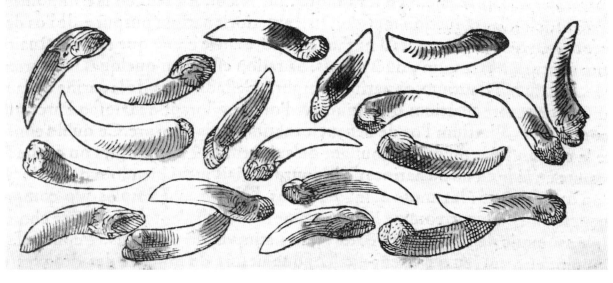

ONGLE AROMATIC.

Woodcut of onycha ("ongle aromatic") from a 1572 French edition of Pietro Andrea Mattioli's commentary on Dioscorides

Onycha, known in Latin as *unguis odorata*—literally, "fragrant nail"—is bent or curved like the claw of a large animal and ringed like a tree. It looks just look like an ordinary shell until you understand its history and that it was called for as part of the famous Ketoret incense from the Old Testament.

The instructions given to Moses for compounding the holy incense were as follow:— "Take unto thee sweet spices, stacte, and onycha, and galbanum; these sweet spices with pure frankincense; of each shall there be a like weight: and thou shalt make it a perfume, a confection after the art of the apothecary (or *perfumer*), tempered together pure and holy." [Exodus 30.34–35] The word *perfumer* occurs in some of the translations instead of that of *apothecary*, which is easily accounted for by the fact that in those times both callings were combined in one.
—Rimmel, *The Book of Perfumes*, 1865

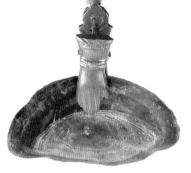

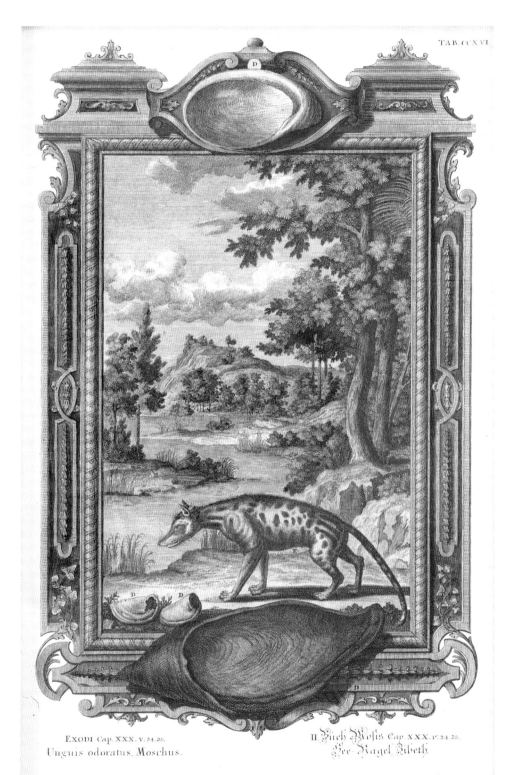

TAB. CCXVI.

EXODI Cap. XXX. v. 34. 35.
Unguis odoratus, Moschus.

II Buch Mosis Cap XXX. v. 34. 35.
Der Nagel Zibeth.

G. D. Heuman sculps.

A Swiss engraving of 1731 showing onycha shells that closely resemble the large shell in the Aftel Archive's exhibit (above). A civet is also pictured.

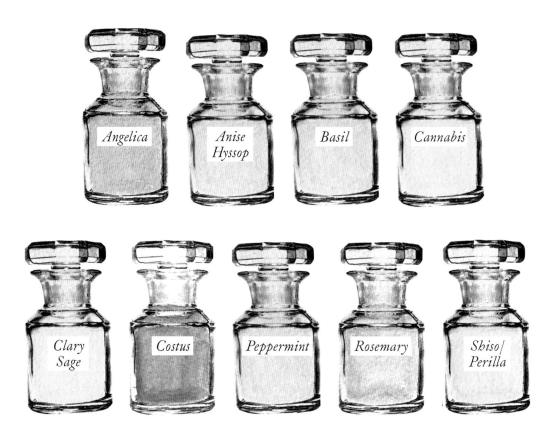

Angelica

Anise Hyssop

Basil

Cannabis

Clary Sage

Costus

Peppermint

Rosemary

Shiso/Perilla

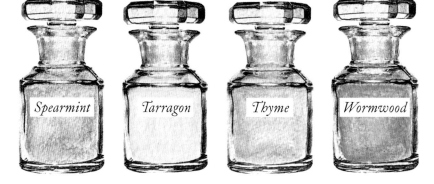

Spearmint

Tarragon

Thyme

Wormwood

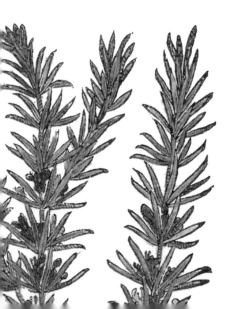

25
The Herbal Family

Science has proved to us by analysis the medicinal value of many common herbs of our fields and hedges, the virtues of which were revealed to our remote ancestors by observation and experience, aided perhaps by an unconscious belief in what came to be formulated in the 16th century as the Doctrine of Signatures. This belief, which seems to have existed, at any rate in embryo, from earliest times, recognized in the external all the signs of the internal. Applied to plants, the doctrine professed to be able to gauge from the appearance of a root or leaf or flower, and how and where it grew, its otherwise concealed curative principles.
—Mrs. C. F. Leyel, *The Magic of Herbs*, 1926

Because of our deep connection to herbs for both cooking and medicine, their aromas are familiar and comforting. Herbs are aromatic leaves that are a part of our collective imagination, intertwining magic, medicine, and food. Unlike most spices, with their aura of the faraway and the exotic, herbs tend to make us think of home, where some of us indeed grow them. Their essences have an aromatic lightness and remind us of gardening—restorative and relaxing. The aromas of herbs are simpler than those of flowers and are closer together as a group, largely because of the considerable overlap of their most common aroma molecules.

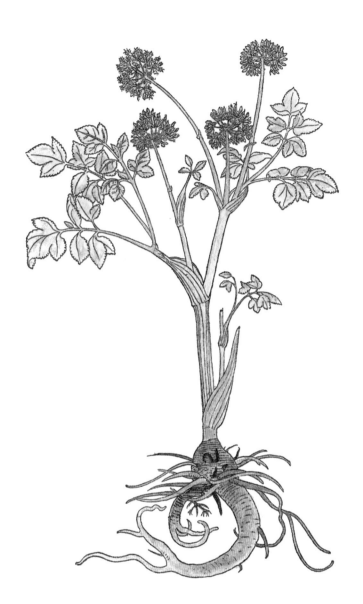

Angelica

Angelica archangelica

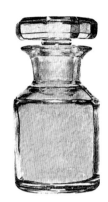

Angelica essential oil, distilled from the root, combines the muskiness of the aroma molecule ambrettolide with greenness. Warm, bitter, earthy, and herbal, with a spicy undertone, the oil is used to make the liqueurs Cointreau and Chartreuse. According to one legend, angelica was revealed to a monk in a dream as a cure for the plague. All parts of the plant—stalks, seeds, leaves, and roots—were believed to be effective against evil spirits. In fact, it was given the nickname "Root of the Holy Ghost." The Chinese, too, have used it for over four thousand years for medicinal purposes.

Available as an essential oil and an absolute

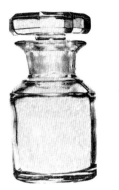

Anise Hyssop

Agastache foeniculum

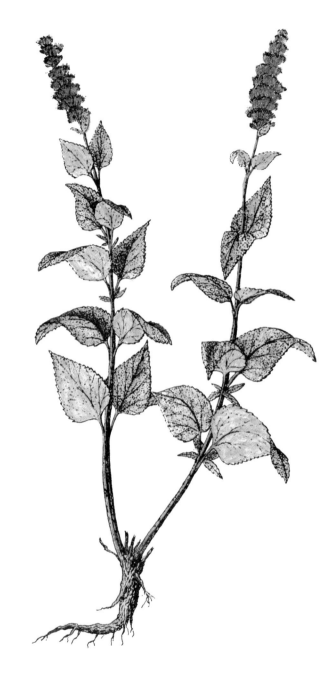

Anise hyssop is a member of neither the hyssop nor the anise family but the mint family. Its mint-like square stems reveal its family resemblance. Anise hyssop's sweet aroma, the perfect marriage of licorice and mint, brings a gorgeous sweetness to the opening of any perfume. The leaves are delicious as a tisane, as are the flowers in a salad. Their tall, lilac-colored floral spikes attract bees, hummingbirds, and butterflies—in short, everything beautiful flying around in your garden.

Available as an extremely rare essential oil

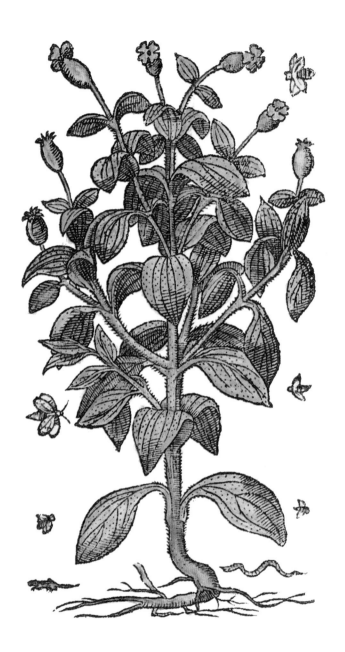

Basil

Ocimum basilicum

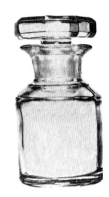

The aroma of basil is green, sweet-spicy, and anisic, with facets of clove. The essential oils from different kinds of basil differ wildly depending on region, season, variety, and stage of maturity. There are more than sixty species of basil, each with a distinct chemical makeup and resulting aromatic facets. Sweet basil, the most common variety, is floral and delicate because of the major presence of linalool (floral). Holy basil contains more eugenol (clove), which makes it spicier, and Thai basil has more methyl chavicol, which gives it more of a licorice facet. Basil leaves have dot-like glands that contain essential oil, but the oil in the flowers is the best quality: if you grow the plant, let it flower and use the blossoms!

Available as an essential oil with surprisingly high odor intensity and an absolute (much less common) that is warmer and softer

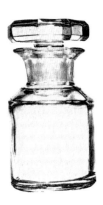

Cannabis

Cannabis sativa

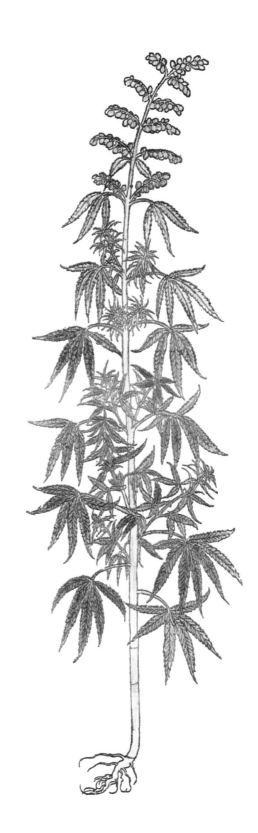

With its intense, herbaceous, earthy, bitter aroma, cannabis essential oil smells like a bag of marijuana buds. The essential oil, distilled from the leaves and the flowering tops, doesn't contain CBD or THC. The aroma is polarizing and hard to blend. Cannabis was used in ancient Egypt for medicine, and cannabis pollen has been identified on the mummy of Ramses the Great.

Available as an essential oil

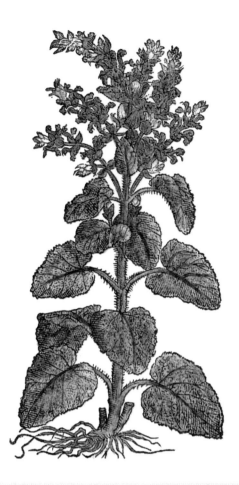

Clary Sage

Salvia sclarea

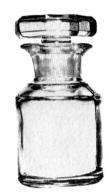

Clary sage's name derives from the Latin *clarus*, meaning "clear," and it was commonly known as "clear eye," because its sticky seeds were used to cleanse the eye of foreign bodies. The powdered flowers are used in the manufacture of vermouth.

The green parts of the plant, especially the flowering tops, contain the essential oil. Clary sage's aroma is sweet ambery, warm, and herbaceous, and faintly reminiscent of ambergris. People find the aroma calming, and it imparts a mellowness to almost any perfume blend. Clary sage has none of the camphorous sharpness of garden sage, because it contains a significant amount of the floral aroma molecule linalool.

Available as an essential oil and an absolute

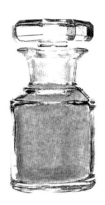

Costus

Saussurea lappa
(or *Dolomiaea costus*)

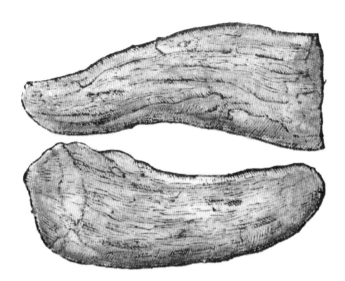

Costus essential oil, distilled from the root, is scarce and extremely expensive. With its singular scent of violets, old wood, and wet dog fur, it has an alchemical effect on every other essence. Costus is very tenacious and diffusive, with high odor intensity, and introduces warmth to a perfume. In a perfume, costus enhances and transforms the blend much as an animal essence does. The violet aroma comes from its beta and alpha ionone aroma molecules. Long used for medicinal and homoeopathic purposes, it was also used in the Ketoret, the consecrated incense described in the Talmud.

Available as an absolute

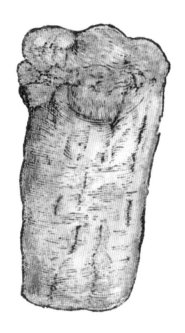

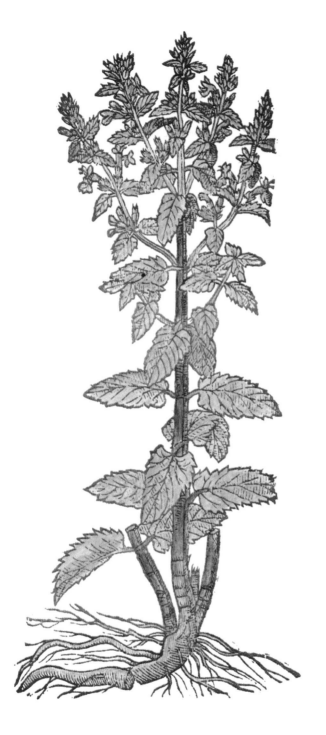

Pepper- mint

Mentha ×piperita

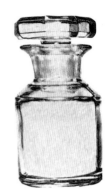

Mint is among the most popular of the herbal aromas, and the most popular mint is peppermint. The powerful and distinct aroma of peppermint is bound up in our common experience of mints and candy canes. Peppermint oil is more than 50 percent menthol, whereas spearmint has very little menthol. Peppermint's fiery bite and pure, refreshing aroma is invigorating, fresh, and cooling, with tangy peppery facets. A tiny amount of jasmone (a naturally occurring jasmine-like molecule in some peppermint oils) helps lend a sweet facet to soften peppermint's harshness.

Available as an essential oil and an absolute

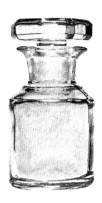

Rosemary

Rosmarinus officinalis
(or *Salvia rosmarinus*)

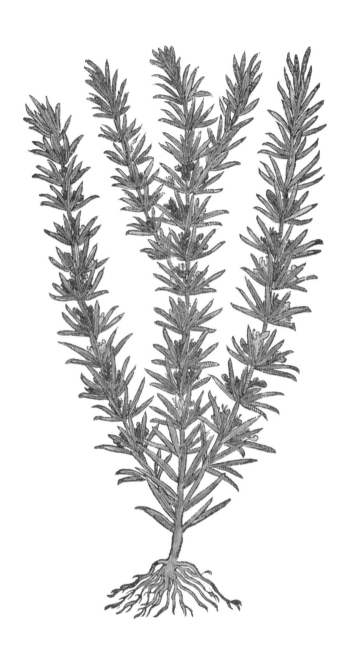

Rosemary, used in European culture since 500 BC, has a reputation for strengthening the memory and is a symbol of fidelity for lovers. Its aroma is bitter and complex, with notes of camphor (borneol), eucalyptus (cineol), and pine (pinene), along with lesser facets of pepper, clove, and sage. Rosemary essential oil is used to great effect in citrus cologne formulas, but it is very hard to blend in more complex perfumes, because of its intense sharpness and medicinal scent. Rosemary absolute, on the other hand, is soft, herbal, and floral, smelling like the plant's little blue flowers.

Available as an essential oil and an absolute

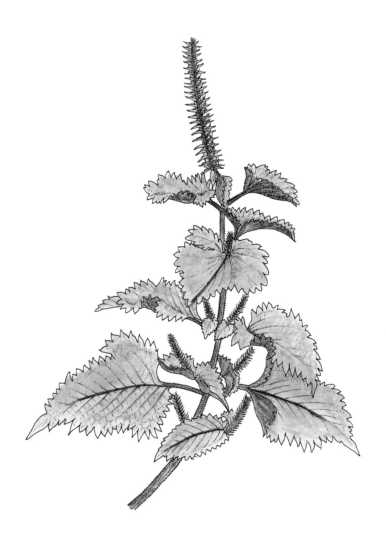

Shiso/ Perilla

Perilla frutescens

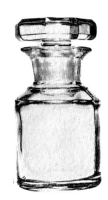

Perilla, also known as shiso, is sweetly aromatic, with notes of cinnamon, cumin, citrus, and basil. The herb is a traditional flavoring in Japanese cuisine, in which it is used as readily as we use parsley. The flavor is slightly sweet and spicy, with a note of mint. The leaves are eaten raw, cooked, or salted and pickled, or used as a garnish; young green leaves are essential for sushi.

The leaves and flowers are distilled to make the essential oil, whose peculiar and pungent aroma cannot easily be compared to that of any other oil. Shiso essential oil is very expensive, and it is very difficult to find a good version, but when you do, you will be transported by its spicy, green herbal aroma. It is extraordinary in its ability to bring spicy notes to floral blends.

Available as an essential oil

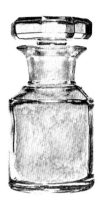

Spearmint

Mentha spicata

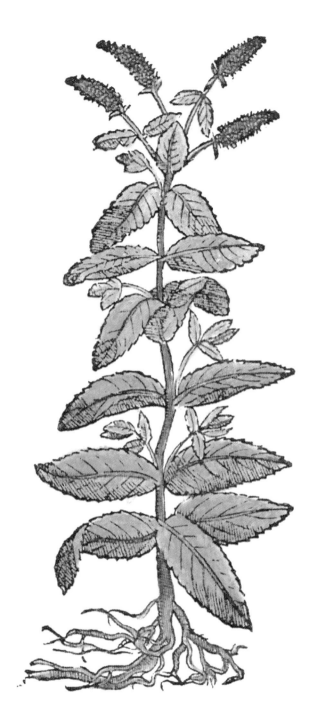

Spearmint only has about an eightieth as much menthol as peppermint, making it easier to use in creating perfumes. It is milder and sweeter, more versatile for both scent and flavor. Spearmint also has fruity facets of mangoes and pears from a tiny amount of the aroma molecule myrcene. The aroma has a cooling and refreshing green character and an almost biting quality. Good spearmint oils have a sweetness to them, while those of lesser quality tend to be harsh and aggressive.

Available as an essential oil

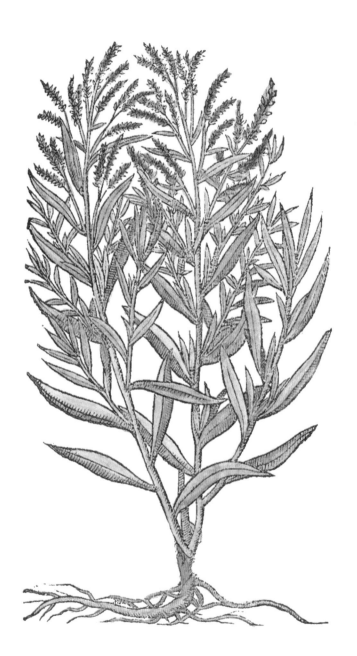

Tarragon

Artemisia dracunculus

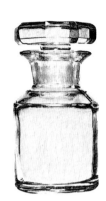

Tarragon's scientific name, *dracunculus* ("little dragon"), seems to have been inspired by the shape of its roots. Tarragon essential oil is my favorite green top note in a perfume! It provides an herbal greenness that is difficult to identify—slightly celery-like, with anise or basil facets—and blends beautifully with almost any other top note. Tarragon absolute, rare and expensive, is velvety, rich, and full of anise facets.

Available as an essential oil and an absolute

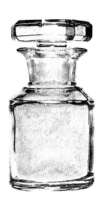

Thyme

Thymus vulgaris

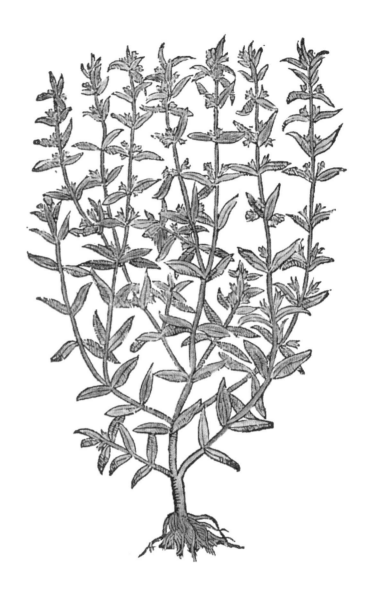

The ancient Egyptians' word for thyme, *tham,* means "strong-smelling," and they used the herb mainly for embalming. In ancient Greece "to smell of thyme" was an expression of praise applied to people whose style was admirable, and the Romans used thyme branches to scent their baths. In the days of chivalry, it was the custom for ladies to embroider a bee hovering over a sprig of thyme on scarves to give to their knights.

Thyme essential oil is warm, dry-woody, and biting but not bitter, with facets of clove and camphor. This sharp, penetrating essential oil is distilled from the flowering tops and leaves of the plant. Thyme absolute smells more like the thyme flowers—sweet, warm, woody, herbal, and soft, without a trace of the medicinal.

Available as an essential oil and an absolute

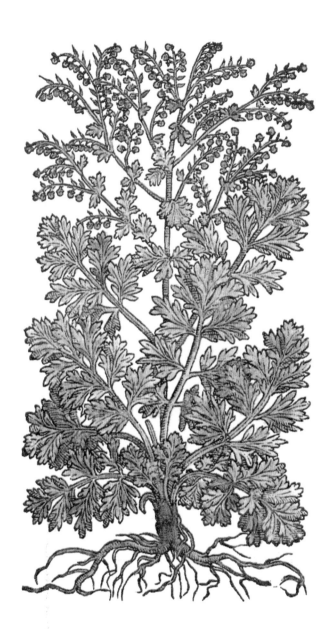

Worm-wood

Artemisia absinthium

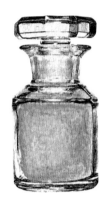

Wormwood, the main flavoring in the legendary liqueur absinthe, is the bitterest herb. In the Bible, the Book of Revelation tells of a star named Wormwood that plummets to the earth and turns bitter the water in a third of the rivers and fountains. According to the ancients, wormwood countered the effects of poisoning by hemlock and toadstools. The dark green essential oil, distilled from the leaves, has a green, warm and deep, dry and woody aroma.

Available as an essential oil

26
The
Rimmel
Collection

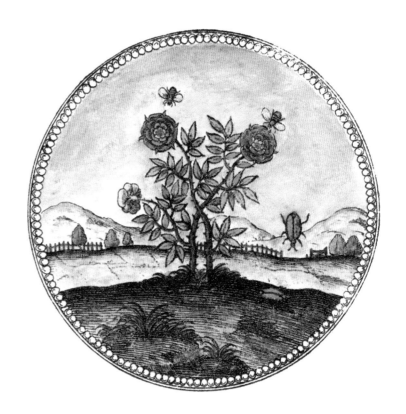

Eugène Rimmel (1820–1887) was one of the most famous perfumers of his time and is well remembered for his landmark perfumery book that has been one of the cornerstones of natural perfumery for over 150 years! His perfume company has gone through various reinventions over the decades and is still around as Rimmel London.

The Aftel Archive acquired an incredible cache of turn-of-the-century essences used by Rimmel's celebrated perfume house; they had been recently discovered in a Paris attic. Many of these hundred-year-old bottles are hand-labeled by fountain pen, and most still have their original contents. Discovering this trove had the excitement of finding buried treasure. I could imagine a person working to create fragrance in their attic with tiny bottles of different shapes and labels—a mini perfume laboratory.

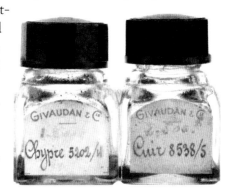

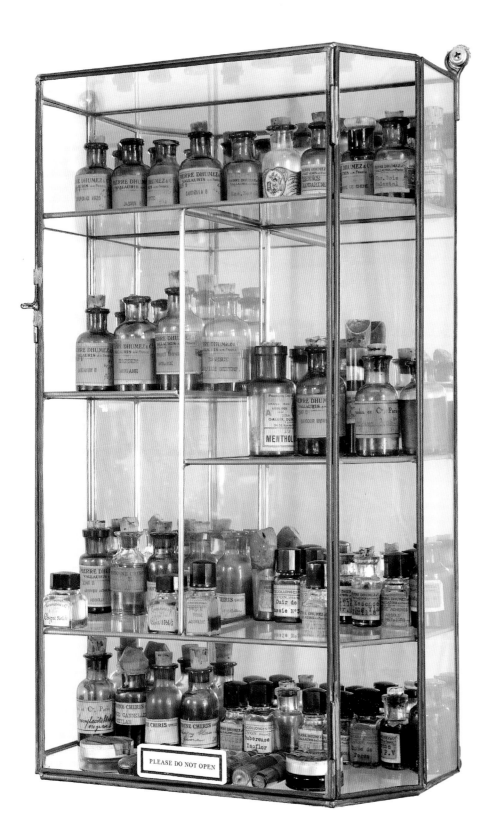

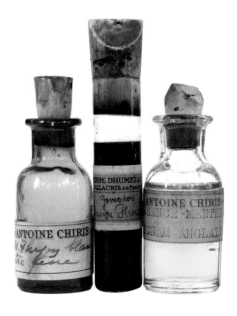

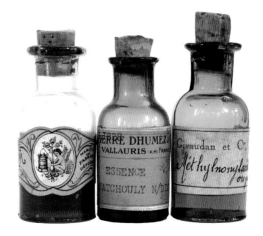

PLEASE DO NOT OPEN

Rimmel's *Book of Perfumes* (1865) contains many of his recipes for perfume and also features his intricate illustration *The Floral Clock* (overleaf).

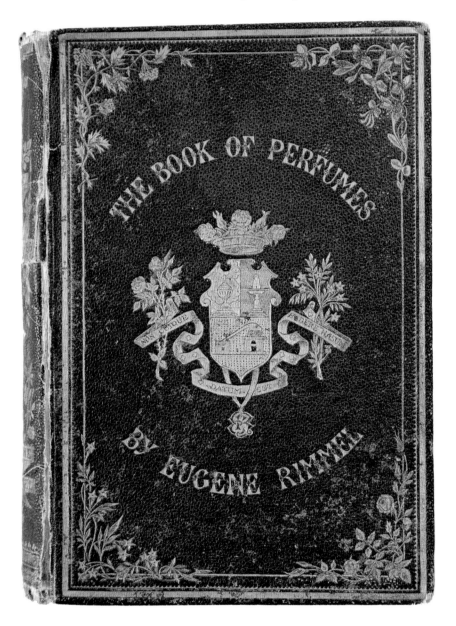

The flower becomes a seed, and its fragrance would for ever be lost, had it not been treasured up in its prime by some mysterious art which gives it fresh and lasting life. . . . Thus the sweet but evanescent aroma, which would otherwise be scattered to the winds of heaven, assumes a durable and tangible shape, and consoles us for the loss of flowers when Nature dons her mourning garb, and the icy blast howls round us. To minister to these wants of a refined mind—to revive the joys of ethereal spring by carefully saving its balmy treasures—constitutes the art of the perfumer.

—*The Book of Perfumes*

Rimmel's Floral Clock

Some Flowers have a stronger smell at sunrise, some at midday, others at night. This depends in a great measure on the time they are wont to open, which varies so much among the fragrant tribe, that it has allowed a patient botanist to form a floral clock, each hour being indicated by the opening of a particular flower.
—*The Book of Perfumes*

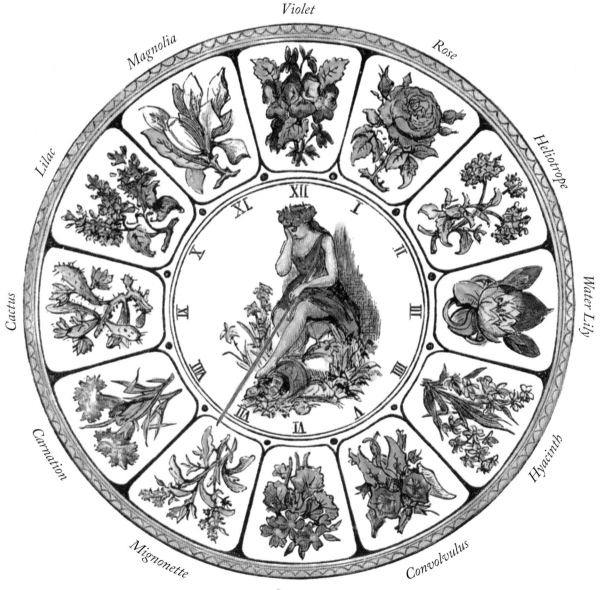

27
Marie Antoinette au Revoir

"A few words on the manner in which perfumery goods should be offered for sale will, perhaps, be found useful. A cincture of red or blue chenille, or failing this, china ribbon, both obtainable at the drapers, will, after capping, add greatly to the tout ensemble. These little matters, trivial as they may seem, are really of the greatest importance, as perfumery is essentially an article of luxury, and requires to be not only good per se, but must appeal to the artistic sense of the individual, both in appearance, general good style, and character."

—An Expert, *Practical Perfumery*, 1896

The embossing plates shown overleaf, engraved with the name of the perfume and the perfumery, were used to stamp metal foil labels that decorated bottles of perfume a hundred years ago. Made of solid polished steel, they convey a seductive heft and substance. Seen together as a group, they have a mysterious symbolic beauty, like rare emblems or charms on a bracelet. The elaborate fonts and small decorations, such as a spade from a deck of cards, whisper the early importance of branding and packaging in perfumery. (The photograph is mirrored to make the embossing plates more easily legible.)

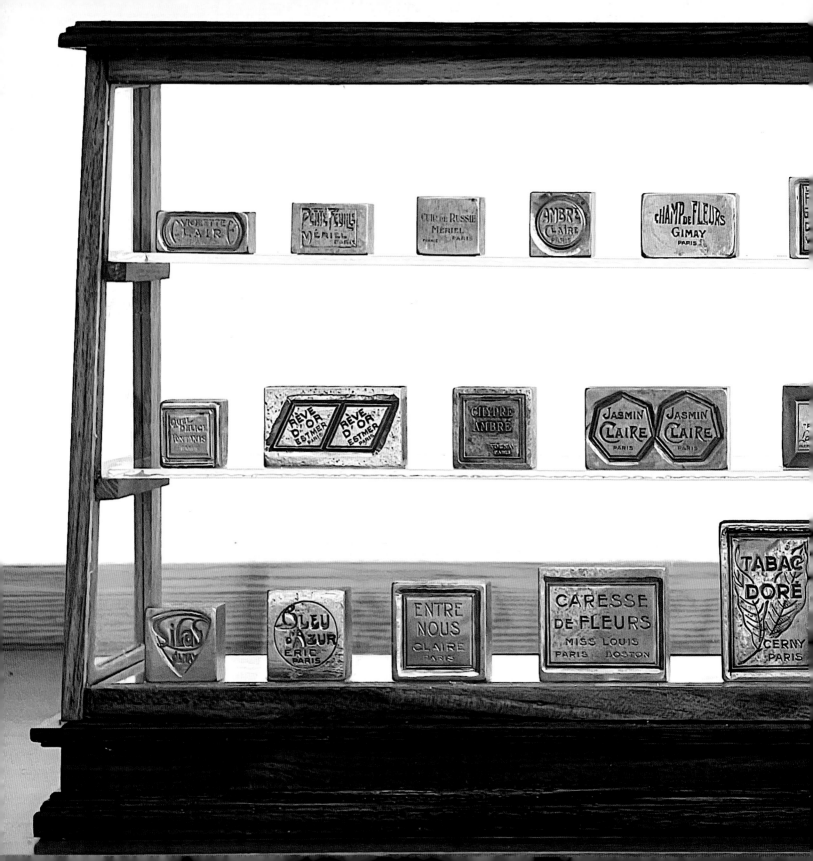

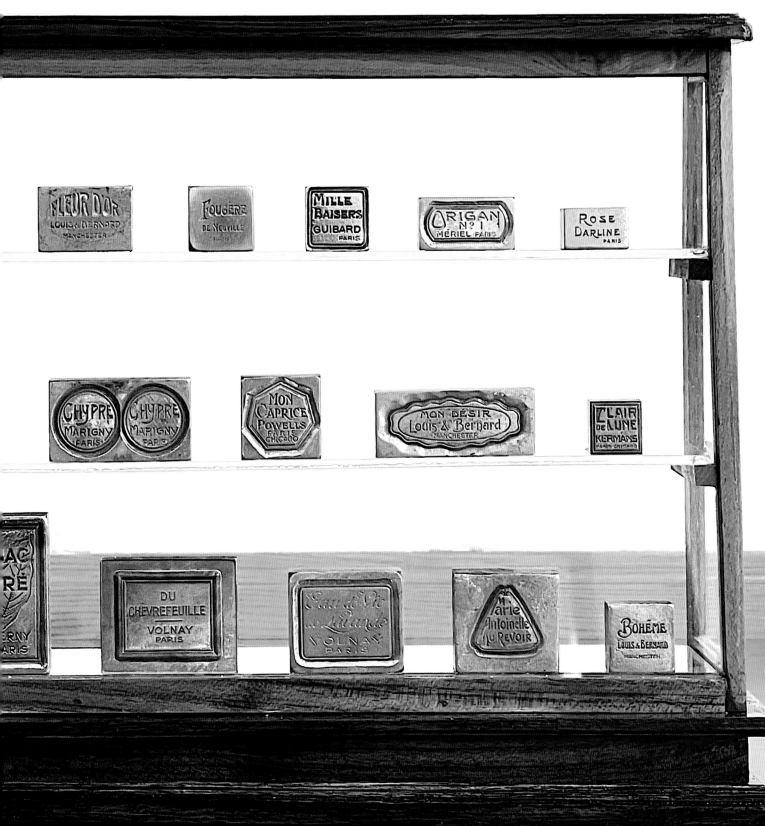

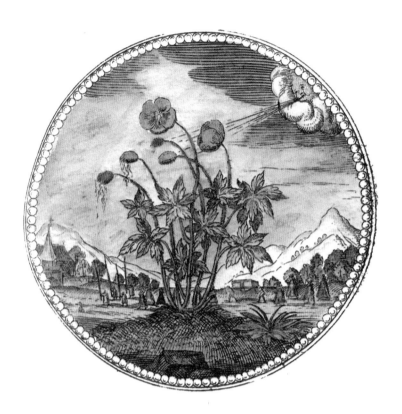

28
The Natural Isolates Family

An essential oil contains hundreds of different individual aroma molecules in varying quantities. A natural isolate is just one of those aromatic components that has been isolated from the others. Natural isolates vary considerably depending on the original botanical material they are extracted from, and they are staggering in their diversity. The natural aroma molecules derived from botanical material are complex. Just like the essential oils distilled from the same plant species, they vary according to the terroir of the plant, and the skill and method of extraction. Some better, some worse.

Natural isolates provide many things to the natural perfumer that essential oils and absolutes alone do not. Natural isolates give fragrances a lighter and sheerer texture in general and can often make them last longer. With natural isolates, the possibilities for creating single floral aromas and floral bouquets become endless. They allow the perfumer to shape existing essences—for example, by using coumarin to add a powdery facet to lavender, adding guaiacol to smoke out patchouli, or creating the exact rose in one's imagination by adding citronellol and geraniol. Floral top notes are in short supply in a natural perfumer's palette; natural isolates remedy this situation.

Early commercial perfumery relied on natural essences supported by high-quality aroma molecules from natural sources. Now, by working with these same essences and isolates, the natural perfumer can return to the glorious early days when modern perfumery started.

Often an aroma molecule smells nothing like the essential oil it is isolated from. For example, you can extract vanillin from clove, even though clove does not smell like vanilla. Some aroma molecules are present in many different oils that smell nothing alike. Soft and powdery heliotropin can be isolated either from sassafras, which smells like root beer, or from black pepper. This fascinating aspect of aroma molecules reveals the vast discrepancy between the various aromatic components nature has put into a natural essence and how the total result smells to us in the end. We wouldn't know what sum to expect from looking at the parts—and sometimes molecules present in tiny amounts can make a big difference in an aroma's identity.

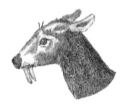

Ambrettolide. A one-of-a-kind botanical musk that is clean and sheer. Isolated from ambrette seed, angelica.

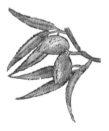

Anisaldehyde. A sweet floral with notes of cherries, hawthorn flowers, and almonds, and a powdery drydown. Isolated from anise, tarragon, basil.

Benzyl acetate. Sheer, fruity, and floral, featuring notes of jasmine, gardenia, and lily of the valley. Isolated from ylang ylang, neroli, jasmine.

Citronellol. A sweet, fresh, green, light rosy floral. Isolated from geranium, clary sage, oakmoss.

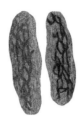

Coumarin. A powdery sweet aroma reminiscent of hay and tobacco. Isolated from tonka beans, Peru balsam, cassia.

Damascenone. Rosy, brimming with black currant, raisin, and plum notes. Isolated from anise, clary sage, basil.

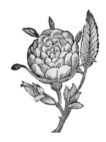

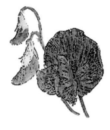

Ethyl phenylacetate. A honeyed floral, like a garden of sweet peas in bloom. Isolated from cane sugar, orange leaf, jasmine.

Gamma dodecalactone. A creamy, milk-like, soft, peachy-apricot, musky aroma. Isolated from apricots, pineapple, osmanthus.

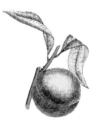

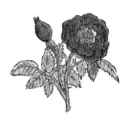

Geraniol. A sheer, fresh rosy floral. Isolated from palmarosa, nutmeg, lemongrass.

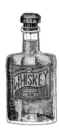

Guaiacol. Divinely smoky, with facets of vanilla and spice. Fragrant notes in common with beautiful lapsang souchong tea. Isolated from orange leaf, birch tar, cassia.

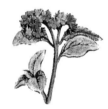

Heliotropin. Smooth and floral, with a smell like baby powder. Isolated from sassafras, black pepper, tobacco.

Indole. Powerful and disagreeable neat, yet when diluted yields a beautiful diffusive, floral, animalic note. Indole is a major aroma molecule in jasmine, tuberose, orange flower, and . . . feces. Isolated from *Magnolia champaca.*

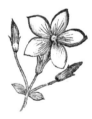

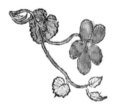

Ionone (alpha). The delicate aroma of fresh violets, with all its floral, berry, and powdery notes. Isolated from *Litsea cubeba*, costus, boronia.

Ionone (beta). Wild violets growing in a forest—floral, green, and woody, with berry notes. Isolated from litsea, boronia, champaca.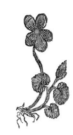

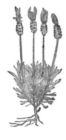 *Linalool.* The freshness of lavender and the light, floral woodiness of rosewood. Isolated from ho wood, bergamot, bitter orange.

Linalyl acetate. A sweet, floral, fruity top note featuring notes of bergamot and pear. Isolated from petitgrain, rosewood, bergamot.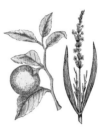

 *Maltol.* Very sweet, reminiscent of cotton candy, caramels, and sugar. Isolated from pine needles, malt, larch trees.

Methyl anthranilate. Smells like orange candy crossed with Concord grapes. Isolated from mandarin petitgrain, ylang ylang, bergamot.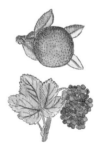

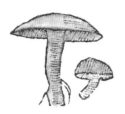

Octanol. A dominant clean mushroom note with earthy, oily, and herbaceous aspects. Isolated from mint, green tea, grapefruit.

Phenyl ethyl acetate. Both floral and fruity, featuring rosy, honey-like aromas of peach and pear, it smells like a bouquet of mixed flowers. Isolated from apple, ylang ylang, beeswax.

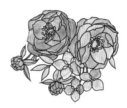

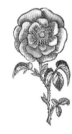

Phenyl ethyl alcohol. A light tea rose aroma with a touch of honey. Isolated from cassia, geranium, ylang ylang.

Phenylacetic acid. Animalic and floral, smelling of heady flowers and civet. Isolated from bitter orange, tobacco, spearmint.

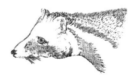

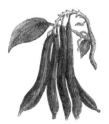

Vanillin. A very beautiful soft vanilla—warm, sweet, creamy, and light, not cloying. Isolated from clove, Peru balsam, benzoin.

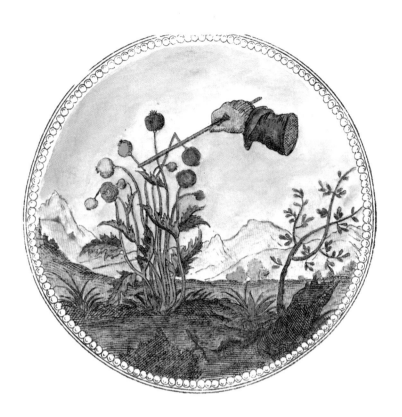

29
Aromatic Magic
Potions, Concoctions, Incantations, and Spells

In medieval times, Books of Secrets were popular compendiums that divulged the secrets of nature, culled from ancient sources of knowledge and wisdom. The information was sometimes mystical and otherworldly, outside of time, and read with a willingness to suspend disbelief. Think Harry Potter crossed with Merlin and *Outlander*'s Claire Fraser. The books, part of the magical tradition handed down from one generation to another, feature a primordial scrambling of appetites and arts that mirrors the synesthetic nature of the senses. Here home remedies are mingled with folk wisdom, traditional knowledge with family lore. Underlying all of it is a love of working with materials from the natural world, most notably a multitude of essential oils from aromatic plants. It is the materials that have the magic. Through the recipes you enter a secret world where you are transformed as you work with them to create beautiful smells, or remedies to heal yourself, or drinks to imbibe.

The Secrets of Alexis of Piedmont

Written by an alchemist and physician, this most famous Book of Secrets is an amazing amalgam of recipes for magic, cooking, perfume, household items, and crafts. The museum has a very rare edition of 1595, "Englished" (via French) from the original Italian edition of 1555. Typeset back when *u*'s replaced *v*'s and *f*'s switched with *s*'s, it demands—and rewards—concentrated reading.

To make one have a good memorie.
Take a tooth or the left leg of a Badger and bind it about your right arm next to the flesh, take also the gall of a Partridge, and rub your temples with it, that it may soak into the skin and flesh once in a month, and it will make you have a good memorie.

For to see wild beasts in a dream.
Take the heart of an ape, and lay it under your head, when you go to bed, so that it touches your head, and you shall see marvelous things, and all kinds of beasts, as lions, bears, wolves, apes, tigers, and other such like.

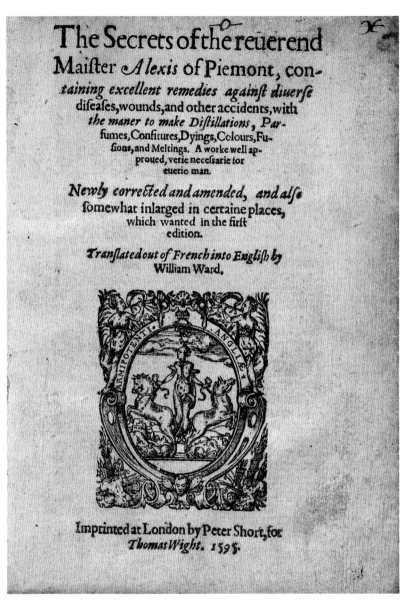

The title page of the Aftel Archive's copy of Alexis of Piedmont's book of secrets

A very good perfume for to trim gloves with little cost, and yet will continue long.

First let the gloves be great, and of good thick leather, to which you shall give a little civet all along the seams; then wash them in rosewater twice: this done, take two parts of rosewater and one part of water of the blossoms of the myrtle tree, mingle them together: adding to it two parts of water of the flowers of oranges, lemons, and citrons, called of the French Men eau de Naphe, and wash them so long therewith they favor no more of the Leather: then lay them on a platter and leave them there with the said water, and poured over with the powder of Cypres by the space of a day or twain. Then give them a little civet with oil of Jasmine, then rub them between your hands, chafing them at the fire, until you think that the civet be pearled and gone through them, and leave them for a while. Then after, rub them well with a cloth, to the end that the civet may pierce them better and the gloves are soft. Then take good perfume to burn, and hold them over the said perfume, to the end that it may pierce and go into the inner parts of the glove and perfume them within. This shall you do thrice a day for 20 days, sweating them each time with a little perfumed water and wrapping them with white linen cloth: then take musk and ambergris, as much as you will, and put it into a tin platter with oil of Jasmine and Benzoin, then anoint them on the outside and not within. Anoint also the seams with civet, and lay them certain days among dried roses. Finally, lay them for a space of three or four days between two mattresses, they will be excellent, as if it were to preserve an Emperor withall.

To make little round apples or balls against the plague.
Take Labdanum, half an ounce, Storax an ounce, Camphor 2 grains, Cloves 15 grains, Nutmegs, Mace, each of them half an eighth part, Damascene Roses, Cinnamon half a dram, Spikenard 15 grains, Musk Civet each of them 8 grains, fine Violettes half a dram, lingnum aloe 4 grains, fine Ambergris 4 grains, Myrrh the bigness of a bean: stamp the Labdanum with a hot pestle, then stamp well the storax, and then all the other things and stamp it with a hot pestle, adding to it every time storax. And roll water until all said things be well incorporated: and then make your round apples or balls.

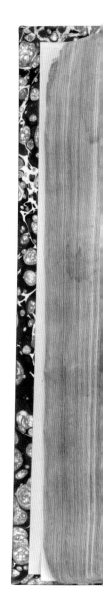

and so keepe it: and when you will occupie it, take the bigge
nesse of a hasell nut of it at a time, with water mixte with
honie, and you shall be assured not to be poisoned: for in ea-
ting poisoned meat after it, as soon as it is in your stomach
there will come vpon you a vomiting, so that you shall bee
constrained to cast vp the meate and the poison together:
but if there be none in your meat, the said preparatiue wil
not hurt you at all.

A secret or remedie not to be stung of Scorpions.

Carie about you of the roote of Polimonia or Polimonium,
and you shall neuer be stung of Scorpions, and if you
be stung with them they shall doe you no hurt.

A remedie not to be stung of wasps or bees.

Take Mallowes and stampe them with oile Oliue, and
where as you annoint your selfe with the vnction, neuer
flies, wasps, nor bees will touch you.

To make what quantitie of strong vinegre you wil.

Take Squilla, which is a kinde of Onion, and take the
leaues off from it, and tie it vppon a thread, and leaue it
fiue or six daies in the ayre. Then plunge it into the vessell
of wine that you will make vineger of, and there must bee
so much void space in the vessell that the Squilla may not
touch the wine being tied by the bung, and lette it hang so
fiue or six daies, and the wine will become strong & sharpe,
and will turne into good vineger.

For one that hath eaten venemous mushromes or Tadstooles.

The chiefest thing is, that he be made to vomit, in giuing
him to drinke oile Oliue, and lie made of the ashes of
the shrubs of vines, or of the branches of a wild peare trée,
with salt and vineger tempred with water. Hens egges
also be good, beeing drunke with vineger tempered with
water. And these remedies be good for any man that hath
drunke plaster, or eaten any thing that choketh, or him to
whome

whom some man hath giuen menstruall bloud to drink, as
wicked women sometime doe.

To be assured, and safe from all sorcerie and inchantment.

Take Squilla, and tie it vpon the principall gate or dore
of your house, and you shall assure all the inhabitantes
in it from all sorcerie and enchantments: and this Squilla
assureth and kéepeth all plants and trées that are about the
house where it is planted or set, from all noisomnesse and in
fection of the ayre.

Against Lightning and tempest.

IN the place where there is tied the skin of a beast called
in Latin Hyena, or of a cocodrille, or of a hippopotamo, or
of a sea calfe or seale, the lightening, tempest and thunder
will neuer fall there, or likewise vpon a bay or fig tree.

To keep that fruite shall not fall before they be ripe.

IF you tie wilde figs vpon the trées in your garden from
the which your fruit falleth, it shall not onlie not fal down,
but also these figs will kéepe them safe.

To keepe that Weasels and other like beasts shall not eat and destroy poultrie.

RUb your poultrie with the iuice of rue or hearb grass,
and the weasels shall doe them no hurt, also if they eat
the lungs or lights of a Fox, the Foxes will not eat them.

To make Flaxe as soft as silke.

Take what quantitie of Flax you will that is good and
faire, and hembe it as readie to be spunne: then take
fresh and reecnt calues dunge as muche as will suffice to
paste ouer the said Flax, and let it be well washed after it
hath remained fiue or sixe houres so soked and couered with
the dung, and it will be as soft as silke, and may be spun as
fine as a man will.

To

Hyppopo tanus, is a beast liuing in ȳ riuets of Nile hauing feet like an oxe, his backe and mane like a horse, a winding raile, & tusked like a bore, and neyeth lik a horse.

The Aftel Archive's copy of Alexis of Piedmont's book of secrets

The Usual
ChymicalCharacters

♄ Saturn, or Lead.
♃ Jupiter, or Tin.
♂ Mars, or Iron.
☉ Sol, or Gold.
♀ Venus, or Copper.
☿ Mercury, or Quick-
silver.
☽ Luna, or Silver.
♄ Bezoar minerale.
♈ ♋ Arsenick.
☉ Day.
♀ Night.
✳ Sal Armoniack.
⊡ Urine.
△ Fire.
⊕ Verdigreese.
⊖ Cinnabar.
⊕ Chalcantum.
⊕ Vitriol.

⊖ Salt common.
⊕ Nitre, Salt-Peter.
⊕ Antimony.
⊙ Oil, of any kind.
⊙ Caput Mortuum.
○ Alum.
♉ Sal Gem.
♋ Cancer, or Crab.
⊞ Sublimate.
⊞ Precipitate.
△ Water.
□ Tartar.
⚴ Sulphur.
♇ Retort.
✠ Vinegar.
✠ Spirit of Vinegar.
♈ Quicklime.
∞ Auripigment.

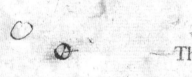

The

LEFT
Alchemical symbols from
Bates Dispensatory, 1759,
another book of secrets

BELOW
The technology of practitioners:
handmade perfume sample bottles
with glass stoppers

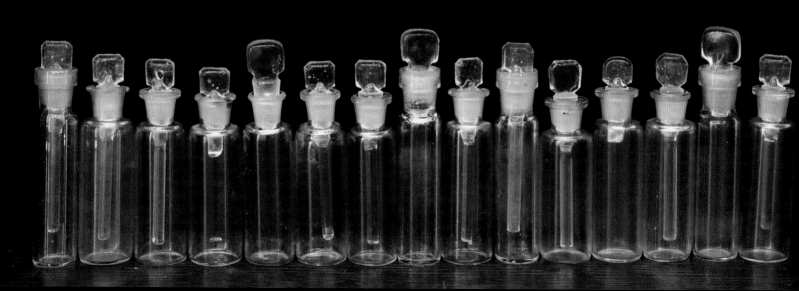

Modern Books of Secrets

The *Techno-Chemical Receipt Book* by Brannt and Wahl (1886) is a relatively modern Book of Secrets. As direct descendants of the ancient Books of Secrets, the more recent versions reveal a vanished universe in their historical mash-up of medicine, culture, and cosmetics. These positively thrilling books promise to reveal secrets—privately stumbled-upon knowledge about how to make things. Recipe books are built on the implicit idea that someone at the beginning of the chain didn't need a recipe—someone who started from scratch: an explorer at the helm, a real craftsperson working in intimate contact with the materials to discover their inner workings and write down the results. Subsequent practitioners pile on their improvements, allowing you insights into the hands and minds of practitioners and craftspeople.

Utterly charming (and sometimes useful), these Books of Secrets extol artisanal work and illustrate the glory of the hand—the appendage that sets man apart.

Recipe books also show the versatility of the materials, which crossed borders and incorporated themselves into people's lives in diverse ways. The natural extracts that were employed in perfumery and medicine were also pressed into service as flavorings. The use of essential oils for flavor is documented in recipes for bitters, cordials, cocktails, colas, sauces, ketchups, cakes, cookies, puddings, candies, gum, and more. A book of the 1850s attests to the multiple uses of essential oils.

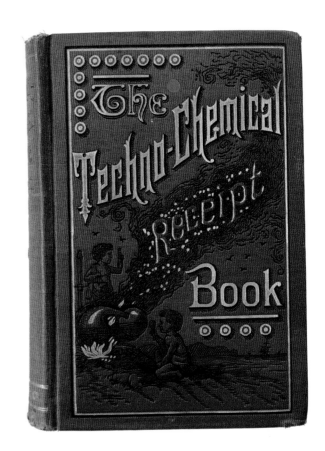

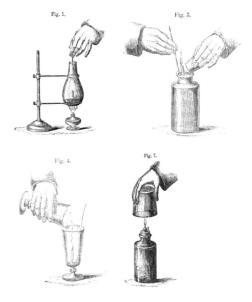

"These volatile oils and scented waters are used as perfumes for the toilet, to flavor the bonbons of the confectioner, or for giving an agreeable relish to the finer dishes of the cook. The oils of roses, lavender, orange flowers, &c., are sold only for toilet use, and for scenting the preparations of the perfumer; while those of lemons, peppermint, cinnamon, cloves, ginger, &c., are employed almost solely by the confectioner and the cook."
—James F. Johnston, *The Chemistry of Common Life*

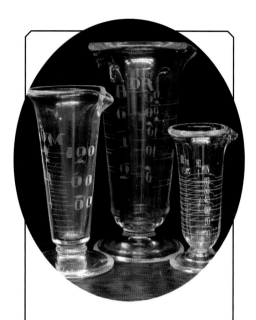

Hand-etched glass labware beakers like these, which measure the ancient units of scruples, drachms, and minims, would have been needed to make the following perfume recipe from The Techno-Chemical Receipt Book.

Ess Bouquet
Four ounces of extract of musk, 2 ounces of extract of tuberoses, 1 drachm of rose oil, 1¼ drachms of oil of bergamot, ½ drachm of neroli, 8 minims of oil of verbena, 10 minims of oil of allspice, 3 minims oil of patchouli, 10 minims oil of lavender, ½ drachm oil of cedar, and 3 to 4 pints of alcohol.

This drink recipe, "Elixir Vital," from *The Techno-Chemical Receipt Book* relies heavily on essential oils for the complex flavor of the drink. The use of cumin oil is unusual, even radical, and indicates a very creative mind at work!

Dissolve 120 drops of bergamot, 32 each of oil of mace, oil of coriander seed, and oil of cloves; 24 each of cumin oil and oil of cinnamon, and 60 of vanilla tincture in 1½ gallons of rectified spirit of 90 per cent. Tr. [tincture]; sweeten the solution with the syrup made of 6½ pounds of sugar and 1½ gallons of water. Color green.

Books about making wine contained tips for harnessing the power of essential oils—including ambergris!—to create liqueurs featuring all the complex nuances of a fine perfume. Full of secret recipes, they explicitly refer to making these drinks as a crossover from perfumery.

It requires a great deal of experience to combine different perfumes to produce any certain required aroma; a knowledge is necessary of the effect produced by perfumes in combination. The mere facts laid down in receipts will not be sufficient for a liquor manufacturer; he must know just what, and how much of it to use, to counteract what is objectionable, and produce or increase the correct aroma. He will frequently find that a single aromatic perfume fails to give the effect he anticipated; and yet the addition of a mere atom of some other perfume may be all that is required. Thus, the flavor of star anise is accompanied by a slight, but objectionable odor of bed-bugs; a very small addition of green anise and fennel counteracts this. Ambergris alone, gives scarcely any perfume, but musk brings it out. The quince has a peculiar taste which is corrected by cloves; the aftertaste of cinnamon is also destroyed by cloves; vanilla has more flavor if pounded with sugar than when ground with it. Absinthe requires the zest of the lemon to take away its naturally bitter taste. These examples will show that considerable experience is needed to be able to blend perfumes with any degree of success.
—John Rack, *The French Wine and Liquor Manufacturer*, 1863

Dick's Encyclopedia

My personal favorite and rather massive book of secrets is the plainly named *Dick's Encyclopedia of Practical Receipts and Processes*, a treasure-trove compilation of sixty-five wide-ranging recipe books from the mid-nineteenth century. It is bulging with recipes for almost every situation life could throw at you, often accompanied by entertaining comments. Here are a few examples.

Friar's Balsam, or Jesuit's Drops
Take gum benzoin, 6 ounces; strained storax, 2 ounces; pulverized aloes and myrrh, each ½ ounce; balsam Peru, one ounce; balsam tolu, 2 ounces; extract of licorice, 2 ounces; alcohol, 2 quarts. Let it stand for 2 weeks, with occasional agitation, and filter the whole through paper. A good application for wounds and cuts; and as such was very effectual in the hands of the old friars. Internally, it is stimulant, expectorant, and anti-spasmodic, and is useful in asthma, catarrh, consumption, and languid circulation. Dose, ½ a drachm on loaf sugar.

Essence of Peppermint
Oil of peppermint, 1 ounce; herb peppermint, ½ ounce; spirit of wine, 1 pint. Digest for a week, or until sufficiently colored. Palish green, and very strong of the peppermint. Essence of peppermint is not conceived to be good by the ignorant unless it has a pale tint of green, which they presume is a proof of its being genuine. The most harmless way is to steep a little of the green peppermint in the spirit for this purpose (as above), or if this is not at hand, a little parsley will do equally as well, and in fact improve the flavor.

Universal Wound Balsam
Gum benzoin, in powder, 6 ounces; balsam of tolu, in powder, 3 ounces; gum storax, 2 ounces; frankincense, in powder, 2 ounces; gum myrrh, in powder, 2 ounces; socotrine aloes, in powder, 3 ounces; alcohol, 1 gallon. Mix them all together and put them in a digester, and give them a gentle heat for three or four days; then strain. 30 or 40 drops on a lump of sugar may be taken at any time, for flatulency or pain at the stomach; and in old age, where nature requires stimulation. This valuable remedy should be kept in every family ready for use; it cannot be surpassed as an application for cuts and recent wounds, and is equally good for man or animals.

The Versatile Apothecary

Long ago the apothecary handled a plethora of disparate products: spices, medicines, candies, sealing wax and candles, paper and ink, and perfumes! Many recipes for such items were featured in Books of Secrets. Apothecaries and later pharmacies were major makers and suppliers of perfume. Many of the hundred-year-old bottles of essential oils that I found for the museum have labels on them saying they were "Put Up Expressly For," say, "W. J. Gilmore Drug, Pittsburgh, PA" or "Newbro Drug Co., Butte, Montana."

Among the uses to which the products of distillation are applied, those connected primarily with the sense of smell possess an interest and importance, especially to the pharmacist, who has, from the earliest time, been called upon to manufacture and sell them, which justifies the appropriation of a portion of this work to their modes of preparation. . . . These perfumes allow of an unlimited choice of ingredients, and a corresponding variety of combinations and proportions, restricted only by that most capricious of all standards—*taste*."
—Edward Parrish,
A Treatise on Pharmacy, 1864

In these pushing, go-ahead times it is absolutely necessary that every one who desires to swim breast-high against the tide of competition (speaking only of our own legitimate trade) must, personally, in order to gain his due ratio of profit, manufacture from the crude substances of commerce, the delicate and sweetly scented preparations that he vends to his fair customers. One thing is essential to success in this branch of the pharmacist's art, and that is, the articles *must* be of the best quality obtainable, and put up in a style both neat, serviceable and artistic. The day has gone by when the old-fashioned 1-oz. long-necked bottle of lavender water, uncapped, and very often with the cork unsealed, brought its shilling. . . . It is a self-evident proposition that this is a trade that should be specially cultivated by chemists. The processes are simple, the ingredients (with the exception of otto of rose and musk) cost little more than the ordinary drugs of pharmacy, and the trouble involved in their preparation is no more than an ordinary Pharmacopoeial tincture.
—*Practical Perfumery, by an Expert*, 1896

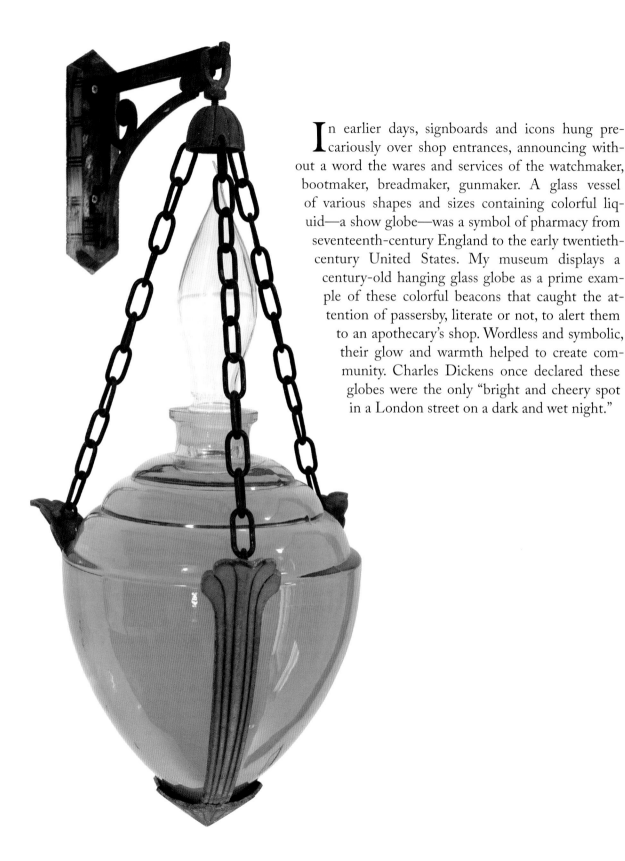

In earlier days, signboards and icons hung precariously over shop entrances, announcing without a word the wares and services of the watchmaker, bootmaker, breadmaker, gunmaker. A glass vessel of various shapes and sizes containing colorful liquid—a show globe—was a symbol of pharmacy from seventeenth-century England to the early twentieth-century United States. My museum displays a century-old hanging glass globe as a prime example of these colorful beacons that caught the attention of passersby, literate or not, to alert them to an apothecary's shop. Wordless and symbolic, their glow and warmth helped to create community. Charles Dickens once declared these globes were the only "bright and cheery spot in a London street on a dark and wet night."

Books for apothecaries and pharmacists also contained recipes for perfume, drinks, and drugs. As you read on, you will see that some of what went on in apothecaries sounds like it was out of a hilarious Marx Brothers routine. The books included some comical instructions about how to fill prescriptions when you can't read them and recommendations not to show up for work in your pajamas. They gave very detailed guidelines about how to retain the customer's faith in your competence when it would be wiser to be worried.

The dispenser who licks the lip of the syrup-bottle, after pouring out what he requires;—who removes any foreign body from a mixture by putting his finger into it, or puts a cork between his teeth to soften it and make it fit the mouth of a bottle, might be compared to an ill-bred person, who, at meal-time, drinks from the decanter, helps himself to salt with his fingers, or cuts bread from the loaf with a knife which has just been in his mouth. He who prepares the dose for the sickly, and often fastidious patient, should be especially careful that he add no extraneous repulsiveness to that which, of necessity, belongs to the prescribed remedy.
—Mohr and Redwood,
Practical Pharmacy, 1849

When a prescription is presented for preparation, the first thing to be done is, to read and understand it. This is sometimes the most difficult part of the dispenser's duty. . . . The writing in prescriptions is often very bad, and the words are mostly abbreviated; moreover, the language in which the prescriptions are written is, in the majority of cases, very imperfectly known to both the writer and the reader. . . . In deciphering the writing it will often be found advantageous to compare the characters in a doubtful word with those most nearly resembling them in some part of the prescription which is intelligible. Should the difficulty still remain, the opinion of a second party, when attainable, should be sought; and in doing this, let not false pride prevent the inquiry being made from those who are capable of judging. Such inquiries, however, should not be made, if it can be avoided, in the presence of the customer. . . . Sometimes a word may occur in a prescription which is quite legible, but the meaning of which is not understood, in which case reference should be made to a dictionary, or other book, in which the terms used in prescriptions are explained, and in this case, again, it should be done without exciting the suspicion of the customer that any doubt exists as to the meaning of the prescription.
—Mohr and Redwood, *Practical Pharmacy*, 1849

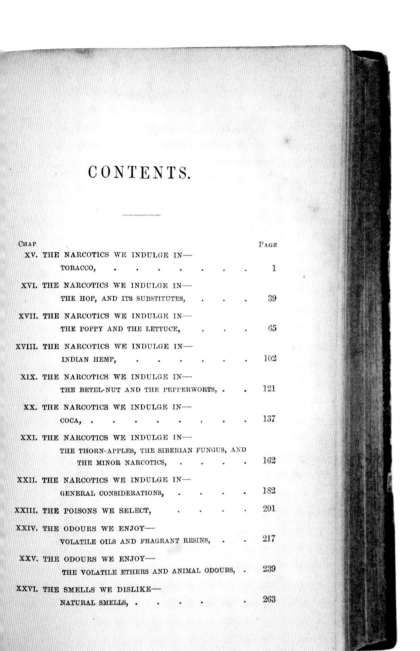

CONTENTS.

The Chemistry of Common Life

The strange bedfellows of narcotics and perfume are intimately intertwined. Perfume was considered a kind of drug for its ability to transport and transform one's mood. The array of botanical materials used for fragrance and drugs frequently overlapped, and the recipe books often included generous amounts of opium. A seminal book about both drugs and perfume, and their intersection, is *The Chemistry of Common Life* by James F. Johnston (1855). From the table of contents you can see that this book is a very wide-ranging romp through man's indulgences in narcotics and perfume. In fact, there are several chapters devoted to "the narcotics we indulge in," wherein the author focuses on the many ways to alter your consciousness with tobacco, hops, opium, marijuana, betel nuts, cocaine, thorn apple, and fungi. Following quickly on this diorama of drugs, the author focuses on perfume because of its compelling ability to alter your consciousness and help you escape reality. One more way of getting high from plants.

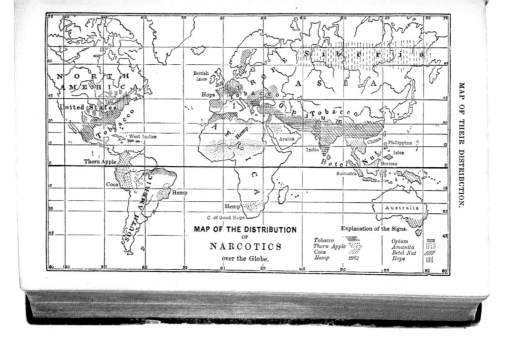

MAP OF THEIR DISTRIBUTION.

MAP OF THE DISTRIBUTION
OF
NARCOTICS
over the Globe.

Explanation of the Signs.

Tobacco		Opium	
Thorn Apple		Amanita	
Coca		Betel Nut	
Hemp		Hops	

Pages from James F. Johnston's Chemistry of Common Life, *1855*

coca to the Peruvian, and tobacco to the European and North American races. The natural craving for narcotic indulgences has in Siberia found its gratification in a humble toadstool.

This fungus has a close resemblance to some of the edible fungi, and is not unlike our common mushroom (fig. 74). It grows very abundantly in some parts of Kamtschatka, and hence its use in that country. It is either collected during the hot months, and hung up to dry in the air, or it is left in the ground to ripen and dry, and is afterwards gathered. The latter are more narcotic than those which are artificially dried.

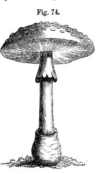

Fig. 74.

Amanita muscaria—Siberian or Intoxicating Fungus.

When steeped in the expressed juice of the native whortleberry (*Vaccinium uliginosum*), this fungus imparts to it the intoxicating properties of strong wine. Eaten fresh in soups and sauces, it exhibits a less powerful intoxicating quality. But the most common way of using it is to roll it up like a bolus, and to swallow it whole without chewing. If chewed, it is said to disorder the stomach.

One large or two small fungi are a common dose to produce a pleasant intoxication for a whole day. If

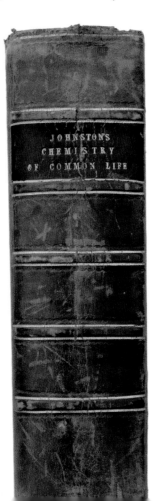

JOHNSTON'S
CHEMISTRY
OF COMMON LIFE

the earliest periods. This is partly shown by the names—*poppy* in English and *papaver* in Latin—which are said to have been given to the plant because it was commonly mixed with the food of young children (pap or papa) to ease pain and secure sleep. In this country, the chief use of the poppy is as a medicine.

Fig. 64.

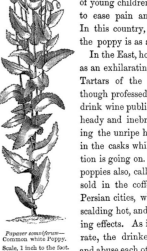

Papaver somniferum—
Common white Poppy.
Scale, 1 inch to the foot.

In the East, however, it is used as an exhilarating narcotic. The Tartars of the Caucasus, who, though professedly Mahomedans, drink wine publicly, make it very heady and inebriating, by hanging the unripe heads of poppies in the casks while the fermentation is going on. A decoction of poppies also, called *kokemaar*, is sold in the coffeehouses of the Persian cities, where it is drunk scalding hot, and produces amusing effects. As it begins to operate, the drinkers quarrel with and abuse each other, but without coming to blows; and afterwards, as its effect increases, make peace again. One utters high-flown compliments, and another tells stories; but all are extremely ridiculous both in their words and actions—(TAVERNIER).

1°. PREPARATION OF OPIUM.—But it is the dried

Acknowledgments

I thank Deborah Needleman for her support and belief in this book, and for her precious friendship. Forever grateful to Julie Anixter for her amazing gift of producing my first perfume exhibit, *Living Perfume*, at Henri Bendel. I am grateful to Chris Chapman for the masterful woodwork that created the beautiful museum display shelves and my perfume organ. I am so appreciative of Chris, Daniel Patterson, and my daughter-in-spirit Kirsty Hume for their love, cherished friendship, and interest in every minute detail of the book process. Thanks to Joel Bernstein for taking the first pictures of the museum when we opened, and for his invaluable photographic advice and his friendship. I am so thankful to Katherine Armer, Sarah Horowitz Thran, and Saskia Wilson-Brown for their dear friendship over so many years. I so deeply appreciate Dr. Clarissa Pinkola Estés Reyés and her grandson Juan "Chico" Dimas for their nearly infinite inspiration and incredible generosity to me. I am immensely grateful to my best friend, Becky Saletan, for her wisdom, brilliance, kindness, and generous love, not to mention early editing and constant hand-holding, with this book and with my life. My son, Devon, and husband, Foster, fill my life with love and joy and laughter—they make everything possible. Full of gratitude for my editor, David Fabricant, for his grace, intelligence, creativity, and belief in my world, not to mention all the hard work he put into this book at every level! And thanks to the other folks at Abbeville Press for their wonderful talent and dedication: Misha Beletsky (cover design), Louise Kurtz (production), Colette Laroya (marketing), and Meg Parsont (publicity).

Index

Page numbers in **bold** refer to the main entry for a botanical essence.
Page numbers in *italics* refer to illustrations.

KEY TO THE COVER

1. Oud
2. Ambergris
3. Angelica root
4. Bushman's candle
5. Rose
6. Oakmoss
7. Onycha shells
8. Frankincense
9. Tonka
10. Benzoin
11. Vetiver

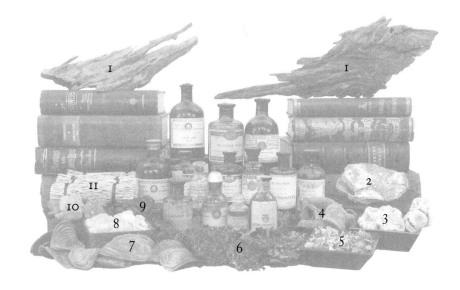

SPINE

The nose of Michelangelo's
David, *cast from the*
British Museum's collection
of nineteenth-century
molds

BACK COVER

A full bottle of Fritzsche
Brothers sandalwood from
East India, early 1900s

ENDPAPERS

The garden outside
the Aftel Archive of
Curious Scents,
Berkeley, California

PAGE 2

The entrance to the
Aftel Archive

Cover photograph: Foster Curry
Cover design: Misha Beletsky

Text and images copyright © 2023 Mandy Aftel. Foreword copyright © 2023 Dr. Clarissa Pinkola Estés Reyés. Compilation, including selection, order, and placement of textual material and images, copyright © 2023 Abbeville Press. All rights reserved under international copyright conventions. No part of this book may be reproduced or utilized in any form or by any means, electronic or mechanical, including photocopying, recording, or by any information retrieval system, without permission in writing from the publisher. Inquiries should be addressed to Abbeville Press, 655 Third Avenue, New York, NY 10017. The text of this book was set in Adobe Caslon. Printed in China.

First edition   ISBN 978-0-7892-1471-3
10 9 8 7 6 5 4 3 2 1

Library of Congress Cataloging-in-Publication Data available upon request

For bulk and premium sales and for text adoption procedures, write to Customer Service Manager, Abbeville Press, 655 Third Avenue, New York, NY 10017, or call 1-800-ARTBOOK.

Visit Abbeville Press online at www.abbeville.com.

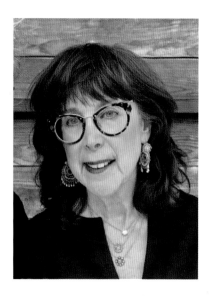

Mandy Aftel is a preeminent artisan perfumer, educator, and author on natural fragrance and flavor. As the founder of Aftelier Perfumes, she has been hailed as one of the fragrance industry's "most prolific talents" by *Vogue* and an "angel of alchemy" by *Vanity Fair*, and listed as one of the top seven bespoke perfumers in the world by *Forbes*. She is a founding adviser of the Institute for Art and Olfaction, which has created the Aftel Award for Handmade Perfume in her honor. In 2022 the IAO awarded her the Septimus Piesse Visionary Award for her lifetime achievements.

Aftel is the author of nine books, including *The Art of Flavor: Practices and Principles for Creating Delicious Food* (Riverhead Books, 2017, with two-Michelin-star chef Daniel Patterson), *Fragrant: The Secret Life of Scent* (Riverhead Books, 2014, Perfume Plume award for writing), *Essence and Alchemy: A Natural History of Perfume* (FSG, 2001, fourteen foreign editions, Richard B. Solomon Award from the Sense of Smell Institute), *Scents and Sensibilities: Creating Solid Perfumes for Well-Being* (Gibbs Smith, 2005), and *Aroma: The Magic of Essential Oils in Food and Fragrance* (Artisan Books, 2004, with Daniel Patterson).

In 2017, she created the Aftel Archive of Curious Scents in Berkeley, California—the only museum in the world dedicated to the history and experience of natural fragrance, showcasing her collection of one-of-a-kind-antique artifacts. It has received thousands of visitors and been covered in *T: The New York Times Style Magazine*, *Goop*, *Vogue*, *O: The Oprah Magazine*, *ARTnews*, and *Sunset*.

Visit Mandy Aftel at aftelier.com.